A Heavy Reckoning

War, Medicine and Survival in Afghanistan and Beyond

EMILY MAYHEW

PROFILE BOOKS

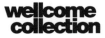

First published in Great Britain in 2017 by
PROFILE BOOKS LTD
3 Holford Yard
Bevin Way
London
WC1X 9HD
www.profilebooks.com

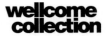

Published in association with Wellcome Collection
183 Euston Road
London NW1 2BE
www.wellcomecollection.org

1 3 5 7 9 10 8 6 4 2

Typeset in Granjon by MacGuru Ltd
Printed and bound in Great Britain by Clays, St Ives plc

A CIP catalogue record for this book is available from the
British Library.

ISBN 978 1 78125 585 8
eISBN 978 1 78283 222 5

Contents

But if the cause be not good, the king himself hath
a heavy reckoning to make, when all those legs and
arms and heads, chopped off in battle, shall join
together at the latter day and cry all 'We died at
such a place'; some swearing, some crying for a
surgeon, some upon their wives left poor behind
them, some upon the debts they owe, some upon their
children rawly left. I am afeard there are few die
well that die in a battle; for how can they
charitably dispose of any thing, when blood is their
argument?

Shakespeare, *Henry V*, Act IV, scene i
(speech by Williams,
the Welsh Serjeant-at-Arms
before the battle at Agincourt)

Introduction

THE CONSTANT OF ALL WARFARE, whatever the century, is the wounding of soldiers. In the play *Henry V,* one of the cultural cornerstones of British national identity, Shakespeare introduces a single character whose function is to do nothing other than remind the audience in raw and brutal terms exactly what casualty in warfare means for the dying, the dead and their dependants. Serjeant Michael Williams is an ordinary soldier whose simple voice articulates not only his fears about wounding but also deep misgivings about the likely costs of a military campaign portrayed in the rest of the play as honourable. It is his remonstration with the warrior king Henry that gives this book its title and provides its epigraph. We never find out what happened to Williams – whether he lived or died crying for a surgeon – but he, like Shakespeare, knew that to be a casualty from a battle like Agincourt in 1415 was almost certainly to be dead.[1]

But not always. This is a book about what happens to those wounded who somehow do not die on the battlefield. It is about the moment and the point of their wounding and what comes afterwards that ensures their survival. Times, weapons, battlefields all change, but for those who somehow do not die, the moment of their wounding – when their power is snatched away and replaced with chaos, dependency and pain – is the same across the centuries. In that moment, no matter how much the soldier has sought to prepare for the possibility of casualty, everything changes at the most fundamental levels of human existence and function. One question fights its way to the forefront of the casualty's brain as they fall: what is happening to me? In the seconds or moments before help or death arrives, their brain struggles to provide some answers.

The immediate response of a soldier in the seconds after wounding is to rediscover what time it is. Being certain of the time tells them whether or how long they have been unconscious. Knowing when it is helps them remember where they are and allows them to plan their survival. But Time itself has transformed as they fall, fragmenting and dilating all at once, and getting it back under control can be hard. Few soldiers owned watches before 1920, so many of those who came to the First World War battlefield relied on the position of the sun in the sky – if the sun could be seen – to tell them that they had lain unconscious for hours, as men around them faded and died, as others lay paralysed watching and willing them to wake up. A soldier at the Somme managed to lift himself up from the mud of the shell hole where he had fallen to find white beads scattered around him. Time passed in some form – minutes or seconds, he never knew which – while he worked out that they were teeth, and that his jaw had been smashed open by a shell and he lay among the fragments of his own face. No soldier in the twenty-first century is without some kind of watch, where time and place can be told in the light or dark, but only if the device is undamaged and there is no crack in the face or fracturing of pixels distorting its output, blood clotting in its cells. Then the owner of the broken watch or phone is no better than their comrade in a muddy shell hole a century earlier, craving certainty, relying on daylight or its absence, prepared to accept even the vaguest hint from the world around them.

Sound, like time, becomes deranged after wounding. Soldiers lie and listen to the sound of their own blood being pumped around their bodies, or drum-dripping on to their uniform or the ground, tiny pats drowning out the sounds of the battle around them. A soldier at the Somme tried to stand and failed, so he lay back down quietly, focusing instead on a gentle, repeating slurp of a sound, like sea surf, whooshing in out, in out. Its regularity gave him a kind of comfort until he realised it was his own breathing and that he could not, no matter how he tried, get it back to normal.

Movement. The ability to move, and to feel oneself moving in time, is crucial. No matter what, soldiers will be desperate to move, terrified that immobility will be mistaken for death. In 1942 an RAF pilot rescued from a downed aircraft awoke to find he was lying on a stone dock wall, completely covered by a heavy tarpaulin, hearing through the thick canvas the last rites being murmured above him. He managed to shift his shoulder, and the tarpaulin was snatched away, a horrified padre replaced by a mortified medic.

Blood. The soldier must find where they are bleeding from and try to stop it if they can, sparking their memory for the fragments of their first-aid training and kit. If they can, and there is much that can prevent it, the soldier lifts their hand and begins to pat along their body to find their wounds. Wounds are always wet, so each touch that finds dry fabric or flesh is a second of relief, before passing on. When one soldier behind a shattered wall after a night attack in Iraq felt his way to a sodden patch on his own back, the moments that it took him to bring his hand from his body to his face, to discover what it was, to taste it in the darkness, those few precious moments of not knowing were infinite and yet not long enough. Hand-to-mouth existence. Finally it was water he tasted on his fingertips, not the saline metal of his own blood. The bullet had struck his water bottle, drenching his uniform. Except that even at the moment when he had almost smiled with relief he knew that there was still a wound to find, because as he twisted to continue his search, it sent pain lancing through him from toes to teeth. Distorted in its path by his water bottle, the bullet had smashed on the edge of his body armour, fragmenting into metal shards, no longer one projectile but several, splattering his spine, his nerves, his intestines, shrouding him in pain.

Pain. Once pain finds its way in the body of the wounded

soldier, it claims its territory, over and over, surges of agony, no ebbing, taking over control of time, place, sound, movement. Pain takes everything from a casualty. Pain will stop them searching for wounded comrades around them, distort their fear and instinct for danger. Pain will make a casualty thrash and cry out, over and over, raw and piercing. The pain of a wound can burn hot, so hot that one casualty tried to pack the hole in his head with snow and mud from a frozen mountainside on an island in the South Atlantic. Pain will draw down enemy fire to finish its job and find more targets. Pain puts those seeking to rescue the wounded in the firing line. From the Somme to Omaha Beach to Tumbledown Mountain to Helmand Province, the first face seen by new casualties has a finger to its lips, shushing them, murmuring them to quieten and calm themselves, gently, reluctantly, necessarily placing their hand over a screaming mouth to stop the noise. Cries turn to sobs of relief, the casualty fighting to regain control with every breath as the medic deals with their bleeding, whispering comfort, protecting them both until the guns find other targets and they can begin to move to safety.

But whether twenty-first-century professional surrounded by their patrol group or First World War conscript, they are no longer the independent, fit young human who stepped on to the battlefield, knowing the plan and their place in it. From then on, the answers come from outside their own selves as their path twists into a distance they cannot see and they can no longer travel it alone. They have become dependent, a human being who is carried, set down, picked up and loaded into vehicles. Around them gather the men and women who work to keep them alive, looking down at them. In what is now a patient's eye line, if they can turn their head or strain to hear, are the others who fell with them, and then their questions become about those others and what is happening to them.

Modern ambulances have waterproof cots, so no casualty on the lower bunk will feel the blood of their comrades dripping down through the sodden canvas of the upper bunk on to their faces, as was often the case in the First World War, taking the sanity of survivors even as they sped on their way to safety. But the design of the vehicle hasn't changed that much, so even today those cots still hang close together. One night in Iraq a young soldier watched his best friend being loaded alongside him. When he did not respond to his calls, he reached out across the aisle to touch his friend's upper arm. The flesh he felt was chilled beyond warming in the close night heat, and he knew that somewhere along the journey, while he had fought to stay present, his friend had been lost. In Afghanistan, no one wounded was alone for very long, but they still felt the shift of time and space before their mates crowded in, before they got going on their first-aid training or a medic began their work, and the whump-whump of a helicopter's rotor blades became part of the soundscape. For others the shift was about fragments, dust, blue sky, a heartbeat under the soil, the dark of a cabin, flashes of tracer and then nothing at all, until waking into utter strangeness, still no idea of time or place, days after the point of their wounding.

But waking. Not dead. In the second decade of the twenty-first century there is a small but significant group of people who have lived through situations of physical catastrophe on the battlefield previously thought unsurvivable. And there are people who have enabled that survival by standing at the limits of life and death and refusing to accept them. For me, this particular group of people are not sources from a history book or a radio interview or a letter home. Many of them are my friends and colleagues, and I work among them every day in a university department that researches military casualty. I may not know their birthdays, but I know the anniversaries of their wounding and I know how many times they have deployed to war zones and whether they plan to deploy again. I know what they take in their coffees, and I have a reasonable idea of when and why they are tired or in pain and pretending not to be. I understand where it is they go in their memory when they turn away from the conversation, look out of the window and fall into silence. When they met me for the first time, I said, I am a military medical historian. I study the history of severe casualty in wartime and its consequences. So, based on that, sometimes when they turn back they ask me another version of the question they first asked of themselves on the battlefield, at their point of wounding. What will happen to them now and in the future – what will be their consequences? And when the medics turn back, they ask me what will happen to the people whose lives they fought so hard to save. And I know them all well enough to know they don't expect – would be offended by – anything but an honest response.

So this book is my answer, the best I can find, to their questions. And while I was thinking about it, I found I had a hard question of my own. What does it really mean to save a life, to bring a human being back from the furthest point of existence before death: what lies beyond survival? As I write these words, they remind me of the oldest of hard human questions: where did I come from? Except that in the case of these new, post-casualty lives, the better question is: where did I come back from? The simple answer is: from a small war fought far away and for much too long. From Afghanistan, where, between 2001 and 2014, 456 British service personnel died and 1,981 were wounded – and for the purposes of this book, being wounded means requiring the activation of a trauma team at the military hospital in emergency response. The longer answer is: from a place where significant numbers of casualties did not die, even though the medical textbooks and all previous experience said they should have. A place where they were officially, and for the first time in military medical history, designated 'unexpected survivors'.

*

The first time I gave the answer that has become this book to my colleague who asked his hard question, I tried not to. I prevaricated, and made jokes about my research being all boring history, and pretended to be distracted by other people around us as we sat at a white plastic table in one of the college cafés. But he's a double amputee who lost both his legs to a bomb buried in a compound floor, who doesn't hide his scars, who's never been inclined to take no for an answer, and he wouldn't have it. So I told him that there is nothing straightforward about what is going to happen to him. Above all, and he knows something of this because he's been researching it for a while himself, the nature of his injury, the one he has survived, has consequences that will last for his lifetime. There are two reasons for this, and they are intertwined and immovable now, in his DNA. First reason: his wounding wasn't just ordinary trauma; it was blast injury. To survive blast injury, a casualty needs not just resuscitation but extreme resuscitation. And that extreme resuscitation, the kind that almost always happens when someone is an unexpected survivor, kick-starts extreme processes inside the human body that cannot be stopped or reset. Although we can bring people back from this point of wounding, closer to death than ever before, something happens to them there that we don't yet understand. Second reason: the blast injury itself, beyond the point of wounding. Blast alters everything: the way cells heal, the way skin scars, the way bones grow back, the way brains operate. Blast affects pain, memory, resilience, every basic human process of life.

In essence, extreme resuscitation and blast injury mean that unexpected survivors suffer and age more quickly than people who haven't been as close to death as they have. They mean that, although we think of this as a very modern war, with the most modern medical technology and skills equipped to deal with casualty, something has happened to the survivors that has a place in the oldest human mythologies. They did not die, they were not allowed to die, death retreated, life held the ground, a pulse beat where there should have been none. But at a price. Death gave way only after a negotiation. The price: life now, less life and of poorer quality later. Myth and science, the deal with death a reality on the battlefield and in the lives beyond.

When I had finished, we were both silent, and I had no idea what would come next except (selfishly) I hoped I had not just lost a friend. A few seconds passed. Then he said, but what we have to remember is that I didn't die. Whatever comes next, I survived. Exactly, I agreed. You didn't die. And we nodded and drank our coffees, and our expressions somehow aligned. He went on. And we know about this now, and we can try and do something about it. Yes, I agreed. We must, we absolutely must. For my friend, who went back to his research office that day, and is still my friend, and for the others.

In the few seconds that passed between my answer and his reaction I stopped being a military medical historian and became something different, hopefully something more useful: a historian of unexpected survivors of severe military casualty. It meant I had to broaden my research to encompass the work of the medics who saved them and of the clinicians and scientists who are racing to understand all the complications that cannot yet be healed, the processes that have been started and cannot yet be stopped. But it's exciting work, because at its heart is a single dynamic entity, with such potential to generate change. The unexpected survivors of Britain's Afghan war are a casualty cohort: a group of individuals sharing a common symptom or characteristic acquired at the same time and as a group, and observable over time as a group.[2] If you think twin studies are useful, cohort studies are the gold standard of research tools. And the Afghan cohort membership is as powerful as they come: all young men, with known medical histories and detailed records maintained from their point of wounding. Everything the researchers will need going forward, hopefully going forward fast and delivering results. But not just for them.

They stand as representatives of something much larger, much bloodier, made up of men, women, children, every kind of human you can imagine. Our unexpected survivors are outliers for an entire global population of survivors of blast injury. Everything you learn here applies whenever news breaks of an explosion in Turkey or Paris or Brussels or Kabul or Karrada in Baghdad or Raqqa or Aleppo. Remember it every time you hear of the legacy minefields and their victims in Cambodia or Libya or Somalia or Bosnia. This is what happens every time a human being, no matter what their background or medical history, is blown off their feet, almost to pieces, by explosions, war or no war, or what is not recognised as a war.

Mostly I'll be referring to the mechanism of injury as IEDs (improvised explosive devices), but recently a weapons expert said that this acronym is out of date. There is nothing improvised about the ones being found in 2016: they are identical, mass-produced by a workforce that moves around to deliver its products where its leaders need them next.[3] Many more, better made but still the same blast wave. Not as many unexpected survivors in countries with second-hand ambulances and nothing resembling trauma teams, but every time more people do not die. And all with the same prospects unless things change. So this is not only part of our national covenant, it is a global casualty imperative.

*

As a historian, I know that we have been here before, a century ago. Wounds inflicted in the First World War by massive shells exploding into humans are very much the same as IEDs and mines that exploded into humans along the roadside and in compounds in Afghanistan. Catastrophic trauma to upper and lower limbs – arms and legs chopped off – great ragged blooms of injury, immobility, bleeding, death close by, closer with every pulse beat, unless someone who knows what they are doing can get there quickly and snatch life back. And then the complexity thereafter and for a lifetime. Which is why this book is mostly (but not entirely) about blast injury that causes limb loss, and why it focuses on Afghanistan, where there were hundreds of these injuries (not Iraq, where there were fewer than twenty, but hints of what was to come). Because in all their stages and across a century these injuries are the greatest numerical and medical challenge.

A challenge where every moment counts, and so when I studied the casualties of the First World War, what I focused on was their journey from the point of wounding all the way back along what was called then 'the carry' and is now called 'casevac' (casualty evacuation). I searched in diaries and letters and journal articles for this most fundamental process in all of military medicine. Piece by piece I came to understand the skill and determination that were required to save a life and keep it saved, under fire, in the worst conceivable conditions. How a little training and an entire hell's worth of experience not only delivered unexpected survivors to operating theatres and hospitals for reconstruction but also delivered the system that is used by Britain's military medics today – refined to extraordinarily expert levels but based on the same principles nonetheless. Move the hospital as close to the point of wounding as it will go, bring clinical capability in all its forms as far forward as it can be sustained. Train everyone to stop bleeds. If they can't stop a bleed, it's not worth going out, medic or soldier. Blood, as Shakespeare's Michael Williams puts it so clearly in *Henry V*, is the argument, whatever the century.

So when I came to research how unexpected survivors came out of Afghanistan, I looked for the same kind of sources that I had used for the First World War. Historians are worried about researching in the digital age: unsaved emails, everything typed into garbled word-processing programmes we can no longer read, degraded hard drives, mountains of low-resolution photographs without captions. Except that it turned out that much of the source material was the same – everyone writes emails when they deploy, but they keep diaries too, and they write poetry, and when they write something important to them, that helps them cope: they print it out and stow it carefully and bring it home. Apart from the biro (diaries from the First World War are usually in pencil or crayon – fountain pen only when there was no risk of the ink bottle being smashed), they could be the same. I've worked with colleagues whose written narrative style can only be described, as kindly as possible, as clinical. But not when they wrote their diary, sitting in the hard sunshine, outside a hospital in a desert camp. Just like their colleagues from a century before, today's service personnel who keep diaries on deployment write fluently, without crossing out, the memories of the day streaming on to the page. Thought to word on paper, handwritten, no need for a spell-check, no worrying about how it will seem, no peer review, no sense of a readership at all, but knowing that they must get it down somehow. And again, just like their predecessors, noticing and drawing comfort from the same things – sunrises, better weather, very dark skies and kaleidoscopes of stars in them, timeless geological features in the distance, animals, mugs of tea.

I never expected diaries, but once I found them, I paid attention, and I looked as I had during my First World War research for handwritten sources. A single reference in a mother's memoir of the death of her son alerted me to another kind of diary: a patient diary. I wasn't the only person concerned to answer the question 'What happened to me?' Medics in Afghanistan, who brought in and treated casualties who didn't regain consciousness before they were sent home, wanted them to know what had happened to them while they slept. How hard the team had worked for them, and what they would have heard at their bedside if they had been awake. So they wrote it down, by hand, in little printed books, that became an hour-by-hour account of their saving, even when in the end it wasn't, from the people who held death at bay as long as they could. Not a medical record but a diary, voices, thoughts to words on paper, from medical staff and, when they got to hear about it, friends who asked to write in them too – those friends who hadn't really written anything not on a keyboard since school but who instinctively understood that this little book was all they needed. Patient diaries are the finest medical primary source I have ever worked with. There is simply nothing else like them anywhere. They let us follow every single step in the journey back, and you won't need a medical dictionary to decipher the wording because these are written for humans by other humans in their own voices, who watch as they endure the first few hours of their survival. These are other answers, invaluable, to the very first hard question.

Questions and answers. Face to face, soldiers and their medics spoke to me with patience and illumination. One of my earliest interviews was with a consultant anaesthetist who served in both Iraq and Afghanistan multiple times. Like all anaesthetists, he works at the head end of patients, so he's good at reading details upside down. As I took my notes he would lean over the desk and point out corrections in what I had written, or make additions, or drew an arrow so that things connected up. He didn't even think about doing it, and neither did I until I went back to type up my notes and saw what sense they made. A military surgeon gave his answers in well-organised paragraphs: out it came, piece by piece, and I broke off from writing to ask if he had told his story many times before. He said no, never, this was the first time. It was waiting there for him to speak it, ready and clear. A physiotherapist, sitting in a beautiful garden that he had built for his amputee patients, talked and talked about so many important things that my pen ran out and I had to go and beg another from inside the rehabilitation centre offices.

I had two particular advantages. First, timing. This book was commissioned by Wellcome Collection in December 2014, as the very last British service personnel left Afghanistan and everyone's thoughts turned from deployment to post-deployment (the official military term for what happens next). And second, I came to them from a good place – one that had already established a reputation for cutting-edge medical and scientific research into the long-term consequences of complex casualty. So when those I hadn't met googled me, they found my personal web page, and saw that I am officially *the Historian in Residence in the Department of Bioengineering at Imperial College in London, where I work primarily with the scientists and clini-cians of the Royal British Legion Centre for Blast Injury Studies.*

It's an unusual post – actually, it's unique. I am the only historian in residence in a university science department in the country, courtesy of an imaginative Head of Department and Centre Manager, neither of whom could think of a reason not to have a historian on the staff. Which is how every day I work with scientists, medics and military medics, engineers and bioengineers, surgeons, geneticists, physicists, patients turned researchers, rehab specialists, mathematical modellers – someone 'who knows how to hit things really hard and then measure them' – because that is the range of skills required to study the consequence of severe blast casualty. I've learned long and complicated phrases such as 'musculo-skeletal dynamics' and 'heterotopic ossification' (and I repeat them to myself at home so I can say them properly in meetings and avoid giving my colleagues a reason to think that historians aren't worth the bother). I've learned about load-bearing and joint mechanics and the bioengineering of hard and soft tissue. I understand that I work in the best place in the world to do this work, and that gives me hope.

And in turn they have learned that much of what they do, the lines of enquiry they follow, started a century ago and was then dropped. That the consequences of this were dire and often deadly for all the thousands of unexpected survivors of the First World War. I've explained why this happened in research seminars and strategy meetings and in this book – and they understand, and are alarmed by how much they recognise as being in play now, after this century's war. And most of all I emphasise to everyone involved at every level that, if they don't follow through, if their work is too slow or is wasted, the consequences will be dire all over again. And this time I'll be sitting at the back, taking notes, for another, angrier book. A different kind of reckoning from this one.

Which takes me back to Serjeant Michael Williams, sitting by a campfire angry at a king, because he knew that after every war, when men die or do not die, there will always be reckonings to make. This therefore is mine. A heavy reckoning. A long answer to a hard question, an account of the human costs and consequences of a small war, fought far away and for too long (a timeline follows). And the reckoning begins, as all wars do, no matter the century, with the point of wounding, at the first moment a soldier falls and what happens to them there while they do not die.

The War in Afghanistan: Timeline

2001: In the aftermath of the 11 September attacks in New York, British Special Forces troops support US strikes on Al Qaeda and Taliban targets in Afghanistan. An interim Afghan government is established and an International Security Assistance Force (ISAF) assembled to bring stability to the country.

2002: The British Army and Marines deploy units to Kabul as part of ISAF, in an operation named Herrick. The first British soldier is killed in Afghanistan. The British contingent of ISAF undertakes counter-terrorism and counter-narcotics operations, provides security in the capital, Kabul, and trains Afghan national security forces.

2003: NATO is given control of ISAF. ISAF's remit is gradually expanded to cover the entire country to support the interim government and the electoral process and to restore infrastructure.

2004: Second British soldier killed. Announcement of large-scale deployment of British troops to Helmand, focusing on counter-insurgency and counter-narcotics operations.

2005: Construction work on the British base of Camp Bastion begun, including a standard tented field hospital facility.

2006–7: Britain's Task Force Helmand, initially 3,300 personnel, deployed into the large, ethnically and tribally diverse province in the south of Afghanistan as Operation Herrick IV. The Task Force is not intended to be involved in day-to-day fighting, but is primarily meant to support development assistance to the Provincial Reconstruction Team working in the two major towns in Helmand: Lashkar Gah and Gereshk. The insurgency grows steadily, requiring troops to move into outlying towns and forward operating bases. From either larger forward operating bases or smaller patrol bases, either specially built or adapted from existed buildings (sometimes forts or more often ruins of compounds and villages), the British forces mount attacks on villages or settlements to clear them of insurgents. At its peak this Task Force would comprise almost ten thousand men and women, on six-month tours of duty, primarily rotating between Camp Bastion and a growing network of forward bases.

2008: Casualties mount, at least six thousand on all sides, requiring the tented hospital to be replaced by a hard-build facility at Camp Bastion.

2009: 'Why we are in Afghanistan' statement released via the MoD web site:

> Our objective is clear and focused: to prevent Al Qaeda launching attacks on our streets and threatening legitimate government in Afghanistan and Pakistan.[1]

The year of the IED. Helmand is recognised as the most violent province in Afghanistan. Britain has 137 separate bases across the area, from smaller patrol bases to larger forts – forward operating bases. For the first time, most casualties coming into the Field Hospital at Camp Bastion are from mines and improvised explosive devices (IEDs), not gunshot or artillery wounds. The British are overwhelmed in the province and gradually hand over military operations to the US

Marine Corps. They continue with efforts to train the Afghan National Army, to create stable governance structures and economic development. Troops continue to operate from forward operating bases to liaise with local populations. Special forces and intelligence assets are diverted from high-value work against commanders in the province to combat those building and laying IEDs.

2010: In the hospital at Bastion, this is known as 'the year of the hammering'. IEDs continue to kill and maim, regardless of strategy, tactics or changes in vehicle armouring.

2011: The worst year for civilian casualties so far. Twenty-seven thousand people are displaced in Helmand Province.

2012: Britain announces it will begin to scale back its military involvement in Afghanistan, handing over to the Afghan National Army (ANA).

2013: Thousands of civilian deaths and displacements continue. Much of the Afghan refugee population that will eventually reach the shores of the Mediterranean begins its journey here.

2014: Britain withdraws the last of its forces from Afghanistan. Camp Bastion is handed over to the ANA, including a scaled-down hospital. ANA casualties remain steadily high. IEDs do not recognise the British withdrawal and continue to explode.

PART ONE

AFGHANISTAN

'What has happened to me?'

1

'Blood is the argument':
The Pathophysiology of Shock

Shock is the general response of the body to inadequate tissue perfusion and oxygenation. This simple statement encompasses a complex pathophysiological process. If progressive and uncorrected, this process will lead to cell death, organ failure and the death of the casualty.[1]

IN ORDER TO STAY ALIVE, a person needs to breathe every few seconds. Oxygen gives every cell in our bodies the ability to generate energy necessary for life to be sustained. Breathing carries oxygen down into the lungs, where it is infused through the finest membranes in the human body into red blood cells that then circulate from head to toes. This is oxygenated blood, and when a person is wounded, its loss will determine whether they start to heal or, in the case of such extreme forces as blast, start to die. Everyone knows that a human being will die if they lose too much blood. This is why.

Blast blows holes in the body that bleed profusely, cata-strophically, oxygenated blood draining out and around them, or inside the body's own cavities without a drop spilling on the floor – going everywhere except where blood needs to be. One of the simplest ways to see if this is happening after injury is by compressing a fingernail. If the colour fails to return after two seconds (the length of time it takes to say 'capillary refill'), then circulation is compromised. However, the test may not be effective if it takes place in freezing darkness or blinding sunshine, where the fingernail may be caked in dirt and gore because its owner may have clutched their hand to their wound in an effort to stem the tide of blood, because they are shocked beyond rational action, because they cannot see, because they are shivering uncontrollably from hypothermia as their body temperature falls rapidly as its warm energy from oxygenated blood drains away. Shock is the condition a body finds itself in when it can no longer draw on the oxygen in its blood, when it is entering the state that will lead to absolute physiological abnormality.

Initially the body tries automatically to reseal itself after blood loss by clotting. If this doesn't work, because it is not possible to clot on the scale required to remedy the damage from blast injury, then the body prioritises its remaining blood and oxygen resources. It shunts what blood it can to the brain and the heart, effectively abandoning other organs, such as the liver and kidneys. Once the body has lost a third of its oxygenated blood, the signs of shock can be clearly seen, but once it can be seen – grey, pale, chilly, cold skin, flattened veins – it is already approaching too late, so in Afghanistan its presence was always assumed in a wounded soldier. In the meantime, the heart races to keep what blood remains moving: human systems are designed to cling on to diminishing fragments of life, obstinately refusing to let go, except that the mechanisms that have evolved to do this can only do so much, and life starts to slip away anyway. Not slipping now, a cascade, surging through the body, smashing anything in its way. Acid from failing organs floods into the system, breaking down the finest capillary walls, so even more blood bursts out. Less blood, less clotting, less oxygen, less energy to breathe in oxygen, more cold, less clotting, less blood – the cascade stronger, faster, deadlier. Other mechanisms designed to save life begin to collapse. Inflammatory mechanisms and the entire immune system go into free fall. Respiratory distress (no more breathing), no more oxygen, almost nothing left to hold on to, life drawing closer to point zero.

2

Scott Meenagh

THREE EXPLOSIONS TORE THROUGH Scott Meenagh's life on 25 January 2011. It was his second tour of duty with C Company, 2nd Battalion, the Parachute Regiment. And, as their recruitment literature will tell you, soldiers in 2 Para are highly trained to foster qualities of resilience and versatility. Paras are tough and Paras are confident, and Scott was no exception to either of these. On his first tour of duty he thought he was immortal. He knew that he would get home with all the assurance of having survived the hardest military environment on earth, and then go travelling through Australia with his girlfriend. And so he did, but then he went back for a second tour, and he found that, however hard he tried, he couldn't see anything good waiting for him ahead when it was over. He could only imagine the worst. Sometimes he sat and even planned his own funeral, and all the while noticed that he had pain in both his legs for which there was no medical explanation at all.

First explosion. A comrade in the distance stepped on an IED and was blown to pieces. Scott's unit was sent out to retrieve what they could – not just the human being but also the expensive metal detector that had failed to buzz its warning of buried explosives. But that was the order. Scott was the point man, as well as the team medic, going out in front of the group, the sharp end, needing absolute control and vigilance. He had grown used to keeping himself, as he described it later, utterly calm for hours at a time. He was good at that, and it was an underrated skill in Helmand Province. Versatility, resilience and calm. He knew where the group should go because they could see that crows were flying down to the spot, pecking at a foot. Less interested in broken bits of kit, Scott wanted to retrieve the human remains so that there would be nothing that the enemy or the crows could seize as a trophy, so he had a bag ready to stow anything substantial and take it back to Bastion. While two of the unit patrolled around them, he carefully filled the bag up and buried anything too small or too difficult to get at, gobs of drying blood and flesh, in the dusty soil. Versatile and resilient: probably not what was meant in the Para literature but no less true for that. Careful searching and packing, into the evening, and then it was dark and he was done and heading back down the track they had come along, five others with him.

Second explosion. Scott stepped on an IED. Its blast obliterated both his legs, gone, nothing of consequence left. It blew jagged fragments up into his arms, burning their way through flesh and muscle. An especially big piece of something very hot, casing or shrapnel, buried itself at the base of his spine, just above his backside. The blast wave lifted him up and then thumped him down on his back, face up, and he thinks this saved his life, because the wound burned into his backside was large and bled heavily and somehow the dirt that blocked it slowed that down and gave him life time. He remembered seeing the sky and feeling time slow down – a final second, long enough to think I've died, and then no, don't die today. Don't die today, because his grandfather had died a year earlier to the day, and he couldn't let his mum have two deaths bearing down on her year after year on the same day. So time sped back up to normal, and he started to save his own life. Utterly calm.

When Scott retells these exact seconds of his wounding, his hands reach up and lightly touch his shoulders, where his tourniquets would have been, Velcroed to his jacket, and in his memory he pulls them off again, hearing the scratch of the tape as he did back then. Somehow sitting up, he leaned forward and over and applied each tourniquet, no rushing, just as he had been trained, and he remembered that, as he did it, it felt so bad, horrific, but he didn't stop until they were all done, one after the other.[1] Calmly. Very few casualties can do both legs, no matter how badly they are bleeding; it is just too hard, and they lie back and hope the team medic can manage it. But Scott was the team medic, so he knew there was no one he could wait for – it was him or no one, and no one meant death – so he pulled each tourniquet tight, one after another. Then he checked what he knew by then were his stumps, but he'd done a good job, and the bleeding was under control. And on the track alongside him his comrades gathered, calling on the radio for him to be collected by helicopter, telling whoever it was at the other end that he had a bad injury but that it was likely to be a difficult and dangerous landing site and they would try to move him clear to somewhere safer on the portable stretcher. So they loaded him up and started to move.

Third explosion. Where there is one IED, there are almost always more, and so it was on the track. Scott's stretcher crashed to the ground, and someone fell on top of him and screams began all around. Only Scott, calm, still team medic now more than ever, began to call out for each of them to tell him what was happening to them. Four out of the five replied. One blinded, one incapacitated, two others peppered with fragments, bleeding. And, worst of all, one silent, the one who lay over Scott, not responsive. Not answering him, except the weight of his body across Scott's a kind of answer in itself.

Calm, holding calm, much harder now but knowing that calmness saves and panic kills as sure as if it was another explosive buried in his brain. Help on its way, nothing more to be done except keep calling out, keep checking on every-one else. Something on Scott's face, leaking from the casualty who had fallen across him and who wasn't moving at all, not a flicker. So Scott lay there, under the weight that he could not yet think about as a dead weight, and he stayed calm and he wiped whatever it was that was getting in his eyes, because that was the practical thing to do. The two least wounded got to their feet and told him they were alright, OK, that they would get him back, but the first thing they did when they got to him was carefully remove his comrade and set him down beside Scott. He talked to them all throughout. Talked about rugby (he always ends up talking about rugby). Talked while he heard one of them calling on the radio for more help (for more wounded), and he remembered hearing the name of his silent comrade given first, and then in the distance the helicopter landing, forty seconds of being loaded on board and then his own silence.

*

When Scott woke up in the hospital, he found that one of his comrades who'd watched him applying tourniquets to his own legs after the second explosion had left him a note:

> Well done, Mate. Above and beyond as always.
>   Your self-treatment was Mega.

Self. A new emphasis in twenty-first-century military casualty. In Afghanistan soldiers were better prepared to engage with severe casualty than at any time in military history, and unless things went entirely wrong, none of them was ever more than three men away from a skilled medic.[2] But first, if they were awake and aware, what had been instinct had become self-aid. Bring a medic, bring a hospital, but above all bring a soldier's own understanding of what he needs to do to his own point of wounding. All British soldiers took comprehensive first-aid courses in the UK. Then equally comprehensive refreshers when they arrived at Camp Bastion. Then shorter and sharper, again, after they had gone to their bases, every few days if it was quiet, at least once a week: reminding them of the main points, repeating their responses, led by their commanding officer. He keeps it simple but this is what he means. *This is what you do, to yourself, to your mate, to me, when the blasts rings out through the air. You are carrying an entire trauma unit in miniature in one of your pockets. Learn how to use it, and don't forget. Make it automatic, brain memory, muscle memory, head and hands. This is what happens when you are blown up,* says the voice of the CO, well rehearsed but still urgently, week after week, because week after week, someone was blown up. *Don't look away when it happens. Remember, head and hands. Do what you have been trained to do and it is much less likely that any of us will die.*

Not that any of them need much reminding. Self-aid, self-treatment and, above all, self-understanding. It's assumed now that soldiers know why the first step is made by them. That most important of all is to stop the bleeding. Two key bits of kit are in their own pocket. A laminated gauze dressing in teeth-tearable foil packs, impregnated with a haemostatic agent (haemostasis: the means to stop bleeding) that does the body's clotting for it because it can no longer do it on its own. If no one is nearby, or if trapped by enemy fire, if they have a spare, undamaged hand, take out this dressing and rip it open. Lean forward, to find the wound site, pack the gauze inside the wound, poke into its depth, beneath the ragged edges of the blasted skin that confronts them, understanding the site front and back, trying not to be startled by the bright redness of arterial blood.[3] Keep packing until the hole is full of dressing, and then press down. Ideally, according to the manufacturer, for three minutes, but the job is mostly done in ninety seconds, and if the fire fight continues around them, ninety seconds is better.

If the bleeding is from a limb injury (which it mostly is) and it overwhelms the gauze and doesn't stop, or it's not from a hole at all but from a stump, then they have a tourniquet, kept where it can be got at quickly, in pockets or Velcroed to the shoulders of their battledress. Tourniquets are made of a length of reinforced nylon strap, about 2 centimetres wide and 35 centimetres long with Velcro segments to hold them in place when they are folded, and they fold down into a neat but chunky rectangle. They come in three colours. Black for the military, orange for civilian paramedics and blue for training. They have a buckle at one end, and a windlass handle to tighten and lock them. They are specifically designed to be used with one hand. Self-aid with Velcro.

Rip them off, open them up, wrap them around the wound, thread one end through the buckle and wind the windlass handle. Tight. Tighter. Tourniquets stop arterial bleeding, if you can get them on. But they hurt as you wind the handle tight; they hurt like no one has ever managed to describe, and they won't find out until they actually have to use theirs on themselves and they will scream as they tighten, with one part of their brain, knowing the bleeding must be stopped, fighting another part that screams *stop the pain, stop it, you know how to stop it. Lie back, let go and let the pain bleed away.* They don't listen to that part of their brain but keep tightening, keep watching and feeling for the blood to stop, and if it doesn't, use another one until it does. That's why Scott getting his on to his stumps without fainting and twisting the windlasses until the blood stopped flowing so impressed his mates in C Company, who had gathered around him, knowing only he could help himself at that moment, and seeing that he did.

It's the tourniquets that everyone remembers from Afghanistan. Everyone came to love them because they worked so well, were so quick and easy to use, and everyone eventually knew someone whose life had been saved by one or two or three of them. It got so that soldiers pre-applied them, strapping them round their legs just in case, before a single step had been taken into the fire fight or along the uncleared road.[4] One kept seven or eight of them on his arms in a private store every single time he went out, enough for him and his mates, in case they were hit and couldn't get to theirs. This is the step after self-aid: buddy aid. Treat their mates, just as they've been trained. Share their own medical kit if their mate's is damaged or they've used all their dressings and tourniquets. Gather round them and keep them awake, keep them fighting back the cascade, if there's no other fighting to be done. Put the tourniquets on what is left of their legs or arms and turn the handle, don't mind the screaming, surely the pain can't be that bad, look, the bleeding is stopping. Look around as they do it, and find the one soldier in four trained as a team medic. He can take over the next steps. (And the soldier who kept seven or eight tourniquets on his arms, so every time he flexed his arms he could feel them clumped there, could still feel them there after he came home, unscathed physically. Still prepared even in a time and place when he doesn't need to be, still in his head in the war. More about that later.[5])

So one soldier in four has even more training than his team mates. He's the team medic, and he's who his mates look for when they can't treat themselves or each other any more, the next step, the next level of expertise at the point of wounding. Scott was the team medic for C Company, so his Bergan rucksack carried even more medical kit than everyone else's: packs and packs of haemostatic dressings, tourniquet spares, antibiotics, painkillers. The longer the war went on, the more training team medics got. Chest seals appeared in their packs during 2009: adhesive transparent round dressings, the size of small plates, that look simple but which treat the gruesome but accurately named sucking chest wounds. Sucking chest wounds happen when for some reason body armour fails and the chest is penetrated by a bullet or a fragment or something hard enough to go all the way through to the lung. So when the victim inhales (blood, oxygen, energy, life), air comes in through the nose or mouth and through the hole in the chest. The air doesn't go straight into the lung but gets stuck in between the outside of the lung and the chest cavity. Exhaling doesn't clear it. Air builds up, and the lungs are squeezed smaller and smaller, eventually reducing the ability to breathe at all. This is the more deadly but less gruesomely named tension pneumothorax. All sucking chest wounds are treated as potential tension pneumothorax by applying a chest seal, which stops air going where it shouldn't and restores full lung function. Some have small vents which allow any trapped air to be drained off and then resealed. Chest seals are no harder to put on than a plaster, except that the soldiers are getting the non-adhesive backing off the adhesive bit under fire, in dust and chaos, wearing those blue disposable gloves, pick pick pick at the sides until they separate (one of the manufacturers of chest seals says 'fine motor skills required to do this simple task degrade rapidly under austere or stressful conditions'). And in the meantime the trained team medic can hear the rattling breath of a body that is no longer sealed up tight. So they practise, and train, and learn the pack so they can open and apply by muscle memory alone.

Team medics train and help out with the weekly training courses and learn more from every case they catch. Not just technical medical training – team medics are the first voices the casualties hear, as they start to work, the first people to start to organise a medical response, to make the soldiers gathered around do something more useful than just shout at their mate – like go to the radio, cover them, do something useful as a group, all for the one who has just fallen. Scott Meenagh said that the truest statement he heard after he was wounded was that his mates had done him proud on the ground, before he was flown away. They did him proud because they had done their training and he had brought and kept them together as a group, even when it was him on the ground, broken, even when they were blinded and riddled with filthy fragments and one of their number was silent. Team medics were always two things at once: team medics and soldiers, whatever was most needed then and there. They picked up their medical kit or their gun, shooting at the enemy, part of the fire fight, or a moment later carefully picking at the non-sticky side of a chest seal with the same fingers that squeezed a trigger, depending on the order shouted at them from across the way. Versatility and resilience.

Like self-aid and buddy aid, the team medic role really

works, so well, in fact, that in time for Afghanistan it was expanded to create combat medical technicians (CMTs), who are not soldiers, who do nothing else but paramedical care for their units. CMT training is much more than a first-aid course. For almost a year trainees learn emergency medical care – trauma care, how to evacuate a casualty and save their life at the same time, and keep it saved along the journey. How to manage the day-to-day medical and sanitary needs of a team of soldiers living in austere environments (austere is a military term meaning dreadful). How to manage a team, how to manage supplies, how to have and be everything that is needed at the point of wounding. Most of the course time is spent with ambulance crews, with medical teams, learning by experience on clinical placement. Everyone knows that this is where they really learn, so some of them do extra placements, on their weekends off, and the ambulance crews hope there will be interesting (another medical word for dreadful) cases for them so they can prove themselves.[6]

And then it's out to Afghanistan to a unit, and everywhere the unit goes, their CMT goes too, away for weeks and months, living in remote patrol bases or out of vehicles (and many of them were women – in and beyond the front line for years already). CMTs are part paramedic, part pharmacist, part general practitioner. For months at a time the CMT will share in everything the unit does: live off tinned rations, wash themselves out of buckets (with water supplies at a premium, so no laundry except their smalls, which they manage to dunk and dry themselves), dispose of their own waste by burying or burning. They even keep an eye on the mental health of their charges as far as they can, watching for the strain, understanding both the vigilant boredom of life as part of a patrol group and moments or hours of vicious, bloody contact with the enemy. Then they lead the process of emergency wound care, trauma specialists, running the scene, organising the team medics, inserting intravenous lines for saline, antibiotics, pain meds. Especially the antibiotics. The no-washing, no-laundry element of a soldier's life becomes very serious at the point of wounding: casualties pick up serious infections from their own skin that prove extremely difficult to shift back in the hospital, and often for weeks or months afterwards.[7]

Soldiers in Afghanistan often signed up for CMT training once they'd done one or two deployments and wanted to find meaning in going back again (Scott Meenagh was one of those). CMT training – like all military medical training since January 1915, when stretcher-bearers and orderlies signed up because it gave them a trade – meant qualifications that helped them make sense of the war they were in, and potentially gave them career options once they came out of the military. Self-aid, buddy aid, team medic, combat medical technician – an interlocking system of care that saved life after life after life. And it isn't just military medicine that has been affected by this model of treatment at the point of wounding. When they come home, a bit more training and then they are a civilian paramedic going out in a fast car, or on a motorbike, an entire trauma unit stuffed in their panniers just as it had been in their Bergan, to complex sites of casualty on roadsides or in cities that, no matter how bad they are, are never going to be as bad as bomb-strewn tracks or compounds exploding with bullets and blood. They are part of a chain of expertise – and it is the expertise that really counts, built on experience of refusing death and the fatality of injury, more than the kit – that has linked into the UK's own civilian trauma network and, since 2010, saved thousands of lives.[8]

*

Here's what this system looked like on the ground in 2009. A unit was returning from a twelve-hour foot patrol in the Sangin Valley to the safety of their operating base. Fifteen of them exhausted, on the edge of nerves worn thin by constant, grinding vigilance, and still some way to go before safety. Then the radio crackled, a long, frantic message: something very wrong when it sounded like this. Another unit had spotted the enemy moving towards them in numbers, preparing to attack across open ground. Little shelter, except a sprawling, mostly smashed-up compound a few hundred metres away, close to collapse but better than nowhere.[9] They ran for it, but not quickly enough, as the crack of firing began as they reached the edges of the compound. Like dragon's teeth sown in the fields around them, the enemy suddenly appeared, standing up in plain sight. The long launch tubes of their rocket-propelled grenades clearly visible as they lifted them to their shoulders and aimed. There was a huge explosion against one of the compound walls, and then constant machine-gun fire. The screams of the unit wounded began almost immediately. Looking around, the team medic could see the CMT pinned down by fire, unable to move to start treatment. He was closer, so aimed for where the wounded lay screaming, more every second. He ran, as he remembered later, like a racing snake, faster than he knew was in him, with gunfire aimed at him all round, turning as he ran, half backwards, spraying rounds in his own wake and somehow getting inside. The only direct hit was on his rifle, smashing it beyond use.

Enough shelter from walls thick enough to absorb the gunfire and time to see that there were four casualties inside: two very serious indeed. One had the flesh from his legs torn every which way by shrapnel; nothing much left at all except blood and a mush of muscle and soft tissue. Two others, also shrapnel, arms and legs but not quite so bad, so deep. And a friend of his, slumped down against a compound wall, blood where it shouldn't have been, seeping through the body armour on his chest. He had been shot clean through, the powerful bullet somehow finding a way through the ceramic plating, which was not supposed to happen, but with enough force to bury itself in the mud wall behind him. Legs or chest? He decided chest was the priority. He reached the man and sat him up against the wall, carefully working from the side to remove the redundant body armour, throw it to one side and get at the wound. His friend, now a casualty, was conscious, knew him and strained his head down to look at his wound as well, slumping back when he saw it. The medic pushed him up straight and reached for the chest seals in his pack and stuck them on, one on the front, one on the back. Face to face, with his friend's blood on his hands, he started shouting at him that it was a small exit and entry point, not as bad as he thought, as it looked, and that he could breathe all right. That help was on the way, that he was surviving and that, as they both knew, if he survived the first five minutes, he was probably going to make it all the way back. That he was going to make it back. He kept shouting as the casualty drifted in and out of consciousness, still bleeding. A friend, but also a medic, there in time, skill and will, keeping him alive.

When the medic looked around, the other casualty with the ripped-apart legs was being brought into his treatment area by his mates. Trails of blood everywhere, the medic remembered, as if someone had thrown buckets of red paint around the compound. A rocket slammed down close by, and two more casualties fell, both with shrapnel wounds. By now the CMT had joined him through the gunfire, so they both worked, yards apart, bullets thumping up the dust and mud around them, one applying tourniquets to the damaged limbs to stop the bleeding from both severed arteries, the other constantly checking the chest seals, to see that the casualty's lungs were still working, that he could still breathe and that enough blood still flowed through and around him. Intravenous lines in, *do you want some morphine?*, shouting against the fighting and the sound of helicopter support, but still two more casualties fell, couldn't treat themselves, didn't move. More enemy standing up in the fields, walking towards them, firing and firing.

The CMT told him that every soldier who could fire back was needed, that he had the two serious casualties under control, that they could hear the huge engines of a Chinook with its on-board emergency medical team prowling in the distance, looking for a landing site. So the team medic put down his dressings and tourniquets and became a soldier again, and turned and fought for a while longer with his reserve weapon, while engineers from the unit blew a path in the rear of the compound to clear a way to escape. He kept firing, not needing to watch as the Chinook pulled in close to the compound, bullets bouncing off its sturdy hull, hovering a few feet from the ground, low enough for all the serious casualties to be loaded. Then away, with huge noise as the aircraft pulled up high and fast into the sky to get clear, and the remainder of the unit prepared to withdraw.

In the last few moments of the engagement, with no wounded, he found himself a team medic again, not wanting to leave behind the signs of his work, because they were somehow signs of defeat, even though this was certainly not a victory. So he shouldered his weapon, and gathered up the strewn foil wrappers from his chest seals and dressings, and the other debris from his medical kit and stowed them in his Bergan, kicking dirt over the thickest puddles of blood, so that when the enemy overran the compound, as they would inevitably do, they would not know how close it had been.

*

An interlocking system. The first steps in the journey away from the point of wounding. Down a track, out of a compound, into a helicopter, hovering feet above the ground. Yet however this part of the journey is made, another has also been started alongside. It's easy to miss in the chaos, but everything about these injuries is also about pain. Traumatic injury is a tangle of blood and flesh and shock and nerves, and pain starts from the moment the blast wave or the bullet hits. The searing of soft tissue around hot shrapnel fragments, breaking of bones, ripping of tendons, bumping, jolting, falling. Survival resuscitation, evacuation – from the scream as the tourniquets tighten, the dragging of open flesh along the ground to a stretcher, needles, adhesive chest seals – everything done to casualties, whether trauma or treatment, is extremely painful.

Pain starts at the point of wounding and begins a physio-logical cascade of its own. A whole soup of hormones, the immune system, the entire nervous system and the patient's own psychology come together in a stress response that is hard to stop. Pain at the point of wounding can kill – a nervous system in pain demands more oxygen from a body already badly deprived of it, and veins already under attack shrink and weaken further. Even without damage to the respira-tory mechanisms, pain can prevent the body from taking deep breaths, and rapid shallow breathing can cause lungs to col-lapse: no chest seal for that.[10] And the more pain there is, the worse all of this is. Even if the sufferer is made unconscious, once pain has started it will come back. Once it is activated, and the more it is activated, the harder it will be for the new life ever to be free of it.

What the textbooks and the consultants tell you is that pain is a complex construct – officially 'an unpleasant sensory and emotional experience associated with actual or potential tissue damage'.[11] If you let them, they will go on to say that there are two types of pain: neuropathic pain, where the nerve fibres themselves are damaged, and nociceptive pain, where tissue is damaged and the nerves in the area send messages to the brain that damage is done and to pay attention to the threat of more damage. Neuropathic pain = damage. Nociceptive pain = danger of damage. It doesn't feel like two types of pain when it is being experienced, but the long words and the care being taken to define the mechanics of pain in precise detail are important, because only now are we starting to understand the entirety of pain. It's researchers working with today's military casualty cohort who really understand about pain being a con-tinuum – not just from the point of wounding but months and years afterwards, because in the military cohort pain starts all of a sudden; it can't be prepared for. Pain at point of wound-ing, acute pain of injury, chronic pain months or years after injury – all part of the same thing, continuously, without end. A continuum. Pain is a continuum.

Starting suddenly at the point of wounding. Ready for the point of wounding, all modern soldiers carry analgesia (the word literally means 'the absence of pain') in their medical kit, alongside their tourniquets and haemostatic dressings. Ten-milligram morphine doses in intramuscular autojects – easy single-use devices, one button, press anywhere on intact skin, just the right amount. In the First World War analgesia wasn't part of the officially issued medical kit (a couple of unwieldy fabric dressings with long cotton ties and a tiny bottle of iodine), but soldiers took it out anyway, among their personal things. Back then, families could buy morphine in sheets in Selfridges and Harrods and send it out to soldiers at the Front. It looked like leaf gelatine and came in leather wallets, and they could break a bit off and melt it on their tongue as required. (Today's pain consultants think it probably wasn't much stronger than the strongest paracetamol you can buy over the counter today, which may explain why the forward trenches weren't encumbered with morphine addicts.) Stretcher-bearers carried stronger morphine tablets in the First World War and, in the next one, ampoules of morphine in solution and syringes. In 2014 team medics and CMTs also had injectable opioids, or a drug-impregnated lozenge on a stick (usually fentanyl), which their patient could put between their gum line and cheek so the analgesia dissolved straight into the bloodstream, fast and strong.

Histories of pain management tend to focus on which analgesia is used and how much of it, and thinking about pain can get bogged down in discussions of chemicals with names that end in '-abalin', '-amine', '-oid' or '-phen'. It's important not to. Because it's that thinking about pain as a continuum that's the breakthrough – from point of wounding to acute to post-operative to chronic months down the line. Managing pain as early as possible is thought to have an impact throughout the continuum. And this approach to pain says that management begins not with a drug but with a question, asked by someone with training and skill: *do you have pain?* Then more questions, even if the patient is screaming, and usually through the questions the patient becomes quieter, thinks about their pain, so they can answer and say what it is like, where it is, and if they want morphine. Asking the question, listening to the answer. Treatment starts by recognising and acknowledging what has happened. Recognition and acknowledgement by someone with skill and experience. Pain is about emotion and sensation, and recognising both changes them, somehow. Then drugs: not an alternative, a range of options. Pain is never good, has no benefit; if you have it, tell it like it is as best you can to whoever asks. This approach to pain says *stop pain in its tracks from the outset, don't let it start*. The more you can do that, the better it may be in the long run. Treating pain at the point of wounding is also hopefully and determinedly treating chronic post-surgical pain weeks or months down the line.

*

Pain, like so much about complex casualty, is difficult to describe, let alone treat. Some of the best descriptions I've ever seen are by a casualty from Afghanistan who has made his new life his research project, as thorough and thoughtfully as any investigator. And he started with his point of wounding. Meet Mark Ormrod, Royal Marine, the man who changed everything.

3

Mark Ormrod (1)

I saw it go up.
A sudden tree of earth and smoke,
like a heartbeat under the soil.[1]

MARKING THE VERY EDGE of survival, the point where the
competition between life and death is at its most fierce, stands
Mark Ormrod. And he stands there on two metal feet, the
metal hand at the end of a metal arm on his good strong hip, the
first British triple amputee to survive the conflict.[2] The human
being who embodies the very concept of unexpected survival.
He should have died – gone into the undiscovered country and
not come back, except he did. And he marked the way behind
him so that others might return.[3] He is still marking the way
back every day of his life, not least by having written one of
the best memoirs of casualty I have read, *Man Down*. Mark
was blown up on Christmas Eve 2007 by an IED. He had gone
as part of the original British task force, deployed at Forward
Operating Base Robinson (known as FOB ROB) on the banks
of the Helmand River. The explosions that were then starting
to smash out across Helmand could have been from what have
become known as the legacy minefields – left over from the
ten-year Soviet occupation of the country.[4] Or it might have
been one of those built bespoke, its echo evidence of the cheap,

durable and effective offensive weapons of choice. By 2009 they would saturate the landscape. Fields full of them, laid into the irrigation culverts that had been used for centuries, and then just enough dry soil kicked over the diggings for disguise. In one two-mile stretch of road, fifty-three separate devices were found, placed at no risk to the bomber, but every step perilous for those who came after.[5] Within a year of Mark's wounding, 80 per cent of those brought into the hospital at Bastion were IED casualties, and a new three-letter acronym replaced GSW (gunshot wound) and RPG frag (rocket-propelled grenade fragment) on the patient notes and noticeboards.

Medics were learning, and everyone who went out from the operating and patrol bases was learning, how to look for IEDs. There could be a small, random pile of stones at a roadside, enough to make a patrolman break into a cold sweat of fear, or badly hidden command wires for a trigger, or simply an absence of local people around, avoiding a slew of newly laid devices.[6] But not always. IEDs might have been laid days or years before. Heavy rain could wash rocks away and cover everything with baked-on layers of sludge, no signs of disturbance, just like those under the ground that Mark trod on as he led a four-man patrol fire-team to observation positions on a low hillside. Looking back, he reckoned he might have walked over the very spot several times that day, but that one time his body weight plus his heavy kit sank just the right depth into the ground to make contact between the sole of his boot and the pressure-plate detonator, triggering at least a kilo of bomb. The explosion was huge, carving an 8- by 15-foot crater out of the hillside and exposing multiple other devices – at least five, and every single one live – all around him.

Mark's body was hurled into the air, the blast wave underneath him destroying his rucksack, water sack and rear body armour plate. Shrapnel got through to tear and burn his back, and everything else was wrenched apart, including his rifle and a tempered steel mortar tube for launching grenades. He had enough time and somehow memory to register a column of black smoke to his left before hitting the ground. Smoke, dust, sand, stone, gravel and a crystal-blue sky above him.[7]

But no pain. As he came back down, Mark felt intense pins and needles in his legs, but otherwise the worst thing was that his helmet had been knocked to the back of his head and the chin strap had got wedged up under his nose so it was difficult to breathe. It must have been a mortar or a rocket that hit him, he thought, and he should pull himself together because anyone in the area would have seen the explosion and known there was a fight to be had or men to finish off. So he tried to turn around and get into a firing position, which was when he found he couldn't move as he should have been able to.

He pulled up the top half of his body to look down to find out why and saw what was left of his legs, rags, bits hanging out everywhere, loose flesh that had once been calf muscles coated in sand, ripped to pieces. There's a medical word for the kind of amputation caused by blast injury: avulsive. Avulsive means that the tearing and the destruction of flesh go on higher up the limb than the point at which the bone is smashed away. This is because the weapon's hard material, such as shrapnel or casing fragments, takes the hard bone, but its blast energy goes further. The sheer, invisible wave of force tears off the soft tissue flesh and everything it carries: muscles, veins, arteries. Propping himself up to a lean on the side of the crater, he heard a small voice in a rational part of his brain saying he should have been bleeding to death, but he wasn't. Later a medic told him that they thought the blast had been so strong that the torn blood vessels of his legs had contracted in shock, temporarily dampening his blood pressure so that the deadly cascade had been stopped in its tracks.

Then from somewhere suddenly, in both his leg stumps, pain. Pain, out of nowhere, and now more pain, swiftly, in his right arm. It must also be injured, pay attention, said his brain; look at it, see what's happening. His arm moved somehow, and he saw above his face his hand, the palm cleaved in two, the skin flayed up to the elbow, the two large bones of his lower arm completely exposed. Left arm by comparison not so bad: just a large piece of shrapnel wedged in his palm, and fingers still recognisable as fingers and still moving, so he could reach across and unclip the strap of his helmet and throw it away from him, so at least he could breathe. Later he thought that he shouldn't have done that because of the other IEDs dotted around him in the crater that his helmet could have set off. But he wasn't thinking that. In his head, time, doing its thing on a wounded human, telescoping back and forth: present – pain, debris; future – daughter, girlfriend. Thoughts racing between what would be his life, flashing images of the waste, pain, debris, death, and all his own fault, stupid, rage at himself, anger tearing out of him.

Everyone out on patrol with him had also been knocked off their feet by the blast, and he could see them all scrambling to get upright, covered in the dirt of the explosion, all suddenly made the same dusty grey, faces and uniforms, and all of them turning to look at him. A particularly close friend made it to his side first, not shouting but using his command voice to quieten Mark, talking over him increasingly loudly and firmly because the injured man was begging him to shoot him, rather than leave him in this state. And then sense started to return as Mark recognised the sounds of the unit gathering itself, preparing to withdraw and take their casualties with them. He tried to take part, calling them together, to focus. A second member of the team had been injured and dragged clear, somehow not triggering any further explosions. Mark wasn't draggable, so, as the others prepared to clear a way for his rescue, one got on the radio and called in the casualty, immediate attention required, send the helicopter to their base. Send it now.

And as the messages were sent, everyone was shouting at Mark from where they stood, not moving for fear of triggering more explosions, but the barrage of voices was constant, keeping him awake, conscious, focused on their situation. Mark responded, picking out the sound of a young, panicking marine close by who looked as though he was losing control.

Mark put all the energy he could into his voice. They had to clear a path to him, to get him ready for evacuation by stretcher when the helicopter got there. They had to do their mine clearance drills, second nature by now; be careful, but hurry up. Take out their probes or bayonets and push them into the ground in front of them, marking clear ground with white stakes and marker tape. Finding a way through. Don't look at him if it helps them to focus. Remember their training. Do it now. Come and get him.

But it was so slow. The air was cold and clean, the dust from the explosion had settled, and Mark noted that there were no flies to swipe away from his wounds. But he was hot now, and the pain and the pins and needles had merged into one and the temptation to drift away from it all was overwhelming, but still they shouted and crept towards him. After ten minutes the team medic got through. Just in time. Mark's stumps had started to ooze blood, and soon his body would lose control of its circulation. Shock setting in. Deadly cascade resuming, death back on the clock. The medic put tourniquets on each limb remnant and dressings on whatever injuries he could see. He jabbed a needle into Mark's remaining intact arm and squeezed the plastic bag to force the contents into the vein: resuscitation fluids and analgesia, life and time.

Then a canvas stretcher, two of the unit picking him up to put him on it and the pain back, pure and extreme. Mark roared out. His right foot was still attached to his leg by a thick muscle, somehow not torn in two by the blast, and it had been left behind as they gathered him up because they thought it had been blown clean off, but it hadn't and now it was dragging behind them in the dirt, all the nerves in the muscle screaming back at the brain. So Mark reached over the side of the stretcher for his own foot and found it with his one good hand, and grabbed it himself while they still bumped along, and cradled it on his stomach, with the muscle stretched and scraped and caked in dust flapping across him, and he kept hugging the boot, clenching his eyes closed, trying to drift somewhere else. A vehicle came forward, and they loaded him up, but there was no paved road, and so they sped and bumped through the ruts. They kept shouting at him to keep him with them, awake all the way to base; even when the vehicle missed a gear and slammed forward, one of the soldiers instinctively grabbing Mark's exposed femur, pinning him in place by his own leg bone. Nothing for this pain in the CMT's Bergan, nothing anywhere.

Then stop, unload, Mark still holding his foot, carry him forward. Inside the base the helicopter appeared over the perimeter wall, coming in low and fast, swivelling round to land as the bay door opened close to the bearer party. Loading, hand signals in the noise mêlée over his head, confusion, but a handover. By now Mark was failing, drifting to black; the very last thing he remembered was sensing the wind from the helicopter's rotor blades and the smell and heat of the turbine exhaust and burned jet fuel, as they carried him into the darkness of the interior.

4

The Medical Emergency Response Team (MERT)

AFTER SEVERE WOUNDING, whatever fluids the body has lost have to be restored, via tubes, directly, all as fast as possible. Breathing must be resumed either by or for the patient, and the death chill of hypothermia that prevents clotting beaten back, toxic cell death suspended. Now, in what remains of the hour from point of wounding, all hands on deck, not on solid ground in a cooled, bright trauma bay, with the patient on a comfortable waist-high gurney. Here, on a metal cabin floor, on a black plastic liner, inserting tubes into a badly damaged human, with everyone travelling at 180 m.p.h., under fire, under threat, on a rapidly moving, vibrating, noise-blasted platform inside a Chinook helicopter.

This is the work of the helicopter medical team, better known as MERT (Medical Emergency Response Team). What happens inside the helicopter is technically known as Pre-Hospital Medicine, but there is nothing pre-hospital about it. MERT fly an entire emergency department and operating theatre, with standard storage facilities, the same bank of monitors as a land-based facility, and a trauma team, all of whom specialise in emergency medicine in real life. It's a four-person team. First out of the bay door are two paramedics (sometimes CMTs, sometimes civilian paramedics, there to experience what only war can give them) who will collect the casualties from the ground and somehow, under fire and a ginormous helicopter rotor, hear what has happened to them. On board, they hand over the same information to the flight nurse, who will administer the team's work during the flight and manage communication between the team and the two pilots up front flying the aircraft. At the back of the cabin is the team leader, who has the final say.

It's worth really understanding just why the role of team leader is so important – not just to the casualty who is being loaded and triaged but to the operation of MERT from the beginning and as a whole. The team leader – the person at the head of the casualty, reading upside down, calling the steps forward – is not what a hundred years of military medicine have led us to expect. For the first time ever, the person at this point – the very sharpest end of the military trauma system – is not a surgeon but an anaesthetist. Only anaesthetists have the collection of skills that can call back a life sent so far off course by casualty. When they use them in war, they are called 'combat anaesthetists'. It's not a very good name, and not remotely reflective of what they can do, because they don't just save life, they sustain it under the most brutal conditions, readying the patient for the next stage of trauma care. Later, MERT team leaders would be emergency medicine and trauma specialists, intensivists, general practitioners, but they all train under a combat anaesthetist to learn their unique, remarkable skill set.

Here's why and how that skill set evolved. As surgery developed, so did anaesthesia. Gas that induced sleeping meant breathing needed to be controlled, which meant putting tubes into the lungs, intubation. Anaesthetists learned to control blood pressure, mostly to depress it so that patients didn't bleed to death as a result of surgical incisions. Polio outbreaks saw anaesthetists move full-time into Critical Care wards so they could manage the patients breathing inside the huge iron lungs. Control of breathing, control of bleeding, this became the job of the anaesthetist, rather than something the surgeon kept an eye on as they went along. By the 1950s anaesthetics had become an -ology, which meant it was studied, researched and improved. There was more practice, better drugs, better skills and, crucially for wartime, better kit. Better kit was efficient, computerised, reliable and, above all, smaller. Compact, powerful kit could eventually be put into helicopters, and with the arrival of portable monitors and ventilators anaesthetists could finally bring in their full range of life-saving skills, just like they did in the Critical Care units, airside.

MERT wasn't just a new collection of skills and kit. It embodied a radical shift in dealing with military casualty, with military casualties. The anaesthetists who led MERT into Afghanistan were among the most experienced military medics at Camp Bastion. One had completed six tours in Afghanistan, and before that five tours in Iraq (which he never described without using the phrase 'the furnace of Baghdad'). Although the worst of the Iraq casualties wouldn't match the challenge to come of blast injury, the soldiers who came into the wards every moment of every day were damaged in ways not seen before: damaged but not dead, the unexpected survivors of their day. Close, intense, prolonged contact with a highly mobile enemy in chaotic urban settings produced bodies torn open by multiple gunshot wounds and multiple fragmentation injuries from rocket-propelled grenades. At hospital, within RPG range and so under fire for most of its time in Iraq, combat anaesthetists in the trauma teams understood that they had the skills to save these lives, but only if enough of them were brought to bear on the injuries all at once, everything that needed to be done at the same time. So a fundamental principle of military medicine changed. No longer one medic per casualty, as had been the case for a century. Instead, as many medics as were available and knew what should be done, with sometimes five medics per patient: all for one, all at once. A new fundamental principle, and what they say themselves says it best: surround and save.

And let's not forget the most important member of the team.

Chinooks are the best helicopters in the world (not a technical assessment, just a personal opinion), although they don't look it at first glance.[1] They are improbably huge and square, named after the largest species of North American salmon, grey-silver and fat-bodied, with small fin sets that look incapable of propelling the fish through the strong Alaskan river currents but which are in fact powerful enough to bring it from the ocean, up river runs and back, year after year. The helicopter equivalent is much the same. It has two rotor blades and three engines, none of which looks proportionate to the chunky grey body mass or capable of dragging it into the sky, and throwing it around, side to side, up and only just down, and then up high again. Yet they are, time after time, month after month, life after life. They land in the tightest of spaces, in an area no bigger than their propeller span or less – once in a very small compound with low walls on all four sides. The blades spun over the top of the walls and the back bay door hit a wall on its way down, so the medics had to jump down to the ground and squeeze round the outside of the helicopter to get their patient. Sometimes the Chinooks don't land at all, just hover a few feet off the ground, and the paramedics have to really jump out and scramble back in after the stretcher and the patients are loaded, but it means the Chinook can get away really fast. Sometimes they stay only two minutes at the point of wounding, but two minutes is all the giant flying A&E department really needs. There is a Chinook display team that performs at air shows, where pilots demonstrate pedal turns, rollercoasters, nose-down quick-stops, spiral descents and running landings to hysterically appreciative audiences. While their crews wave at the public from the open ramp, they remember back to Afghanistan, where they learned all of it, as a matter of survival, so they could get to the point where Mark Ormrod and all those who came after lay, hearing in the distance the whump-whump of their rotors coming to fetch them back.

Chinooks are vital in this, because their passengers only have minutes. Any slower and there is no point, because the patient will either die on the way or more slowly as the effects of the deadly cascade become irreversible. This is what is often called the Golden Hour. An hour is the maximum time that the severely injured – those who are bleeding out their lives because of limb or torso damage – can survive and still be brought back. Much longer and, no matter what is done to them, they will either die soon after or several days later, but beyond the Golden Hour damage is done and sustained and can no longer be mitigated. The Golden Hour needs helicopters big enough to allow for surround and save, and not too far to travel, whether it's Vietnam or Helmand Province or a pile-up on the M4 in the UK. The Golden Hour is more complicated than we imagined when we named it, for it is the time when the deal with death is done. But for the time being, life now, consequences later.[2]

*

When MERT is called out, the crew run from their air-conditioned quarters through the sudden bright sun of Camp Bastion, crunching over the gravel, jumping into the dark of the helicopter. Briefings about what to expect on the ground start from the consultant as they lurch off the landing pad. Last-minute visual checks while they have the space of being the only people on board. The information has come in from the point of wounding, via a 9-Liner report on the unit's radio. It's called a 9-Liner because it contains nine lines of vital information, such as numbers of casualties, how badly they are injured, where the landing site is, how safe the landing site is. MERT helicopters can only surround and save two badly injured patients at a time, so knowing what to expect is crucial. (When Scott Meenagh was injured, the original call was for one seriously injured patient. But the next explosion happened while MERT was already in the air, so when they got there, things were problematic. But they're MERT, so they managed.)

Two minutes out from the point of wounding, the team

assembles in their place at the shoulder of the soldiers of the Force Protection Squad, who will go out and guard them (they pay particular attention to the safety of the landing-site section of the 9-Liner). On the ground, those waiting for them turn away from the downdraught from the huge rotors. Then back bay door down, heat, dust, chaos, blare, as they snatch up patients. Stretcher cases on the floor of the cabin, hands held out through the bay door to help up the walking wounded, as many seated as can be managed, some sent back and told to wait for another flight or vehicles to collect them. Up and away, back bay doors closing on the people still left on the ground, turning away from the updraught, already moving back to where they were before.

Then inside, the medics gather in around the T1 (the code for the severely injured) patients deemed at the most risk. The stretcher is pulled away. The team leader is at the head end, the rest of the crew in their designated places, all looking for signs of life or death or blood. They check on the measures that have been taken on the ground, adjusting drips, checking chest seals, tightening tourniquets. In the case of a really bad high-traumatic avulsive amputation such as those of Mark Ormrod, they add more tourniquets, above the first. At the same time – and this is all at the same time, which is why the T in MERT stands for Team – they fit an oxygen mask if the face is intact, and the pads and sensors that hook the patient to the monitors around them in the cabin. They check for bleeds that may have been missed, that are easy to miss, that can kill just as quickly as the blasted limb – at the neck, the underarms, the groin – packing these as tight and fast as they can ('aggressively', their training manual instructs) with their own supplies of haemostatic dressings. Holding an empty hand behind them, palm up when they need more, knowing without looking that what they need will be slapped into it. Bleeding stopped, almost empty bath plugged, time to fill it up again, according to the team leader who saved Mark Ormrod, even though he had been certain at the time it couldn't be done.[3]

Refilling is easier said than done on the cabin floor, with its plastic liner, which looks like the bottom of a black paddling pool. Veins shrunk flat in greying skin, hopeless to try to dig into them, not enough time or space to beat the cascade. So the team goes deeper, where they know a liquid flow of blood products can be released and sustained, into the patient's bone marrow. The team leader has a drill, a smaller version of the domestic tool, with a switch on the handle that can drive a special needle through hard bone, preferably the shin bone. But shin bones are often gone in the back of the helicopter, so the hip bone or the chest bone or the long bone in the arm, all can be used in the absence of a shin. (In training they use Crunchie bars, because the texture of the honeycomb centre is much like that of human bone marrow.)

The team leader can feel when the drill hits marrow, *zzzp*, less than a second and in, and immediately starts the flow of clear bags of blood products, of fluids – water, salt, liquid analgesia for the pain. This is not just for the wound but because drilling is agony, the patient often bucking up and screaming as the metal hits bone, so it is better if they are knocked out. The next point along the pain pathway runs through MERT. Analgesia is delivered via IV lines for the patient on the floor – pain control for everyone they have taken on board, via injections or nasal sprays or soluble lozenges for those on the seats. Less pain now, hopefully less pain later, and it is easier for everyone on board doing the difficult things. Back to the drill. Bone marrow is spongey and readily soaks up and spreads whatever is put into it, so blue-gloved hands squeeze the bags to push the warmed liquids deep and fast into the patient watching for the normal human flesh tones to return and the grey to recede. (In the field, medics tuck the bags under their arms to get the contents warmed past blood temperature because those are absorbed more quickly than cool ones straight from the cold storage box – a matter of seconds, but this is the Golden Hour so every second counts.) It is tricky to do in the light of a blacked-out cabin, so the medics watch the monitors, which flash hard green around them, listen for the bips that beat life returning, and signal: bath filled – intraosseous transfusion works like a charm – plug holding, move on …

Blood comes first, but the crew must then move on immediately to breathing. Air from the outside is sucked in through wounds to the chest, abdomen, neck, wherever, and gets trapped in the space between the lungs and chest wall. Lungs are fine, delicate things, and it only takes something as light as air in the wrong place to collapse them, inch by inch, compressing and suffocating from within. Decompression can be quick, with a three-inch hollow needle slid under the fourth rib releasing trapped air – the best sound in the world, as any medic will tell you, because it means air is back in the right place again, provided it can be heard as it hisses out. Then the pressure should fall, restoring normal breathing motion – in out, in out, oxygen flowing again.

That might not be enough. Move up from the lungs in the chest to the throat and the neck. *Stridor* (Latin, not Elvish, for 'grating' or 'squeaking') is the high-pitched whistling sound that signals a blocked airway, impeded not by very much, perhaps: a scrap of debris from the explosive or the broken body, a minor wound on the chest or neck, all enough to restrict breathing. If the airway is blocked or broken, the medics have to make a new one: intubation. A tube is lowered carefully down the airway that leads into the lungs, the other end of which is connected to a ventilator to pump the missing air directly where it is needed. The team has practised and practised intubation back at Bastion because they all know you only ever get two goes to get it right (too long without breathing and failed intubation attempts can make existing damage worse), and they have to be quick. So it takes two pairs of expert hands, the team leader and the flight nurse. Some medics intubate lying down, some sitting up; the crew knows what kind of space to make for them, and they start to do it as soon as the team leader has indicated what is necessary. Give muscle relaxants, add analgesia to the lines to the veins as preparation and then insert the tube through the mouth, down the throat into the trachea or, as the training manual states, sometimes directly 'through the large defect' that is the face or neck wound or, as a last resort, through a surgical airway – a hole cut by the team leader directly somewhere, wherever they can, into the patient's windpipe.[4]

Intubation can come to dominate in a process where priorities must be constantly assessed. The team leader at the top, bent over their patient's head, at their throat, which suddenly becomes just an airway, the team leader losing sight of everything but the narrow tubes threading down into the lungs. Except that everything else is happening at the same time: get blood in, fill the tub (it won't work without oxygenation anyway), be careful with the anaesthetic, look up not down, get it right or lose it. All at the same time. There are videos from MERT on YouTube, but they aren't enough to explain what is going on at the heart of it, what extreme resuscitation really means. Blood, air, bone, life, pulse beat by pulse beat, unexpected survivors on the floor, unexpectedly surviving because of the skill surrounding them, the team working ceaselessly, not just chaos captured on a shaky phone camera.

Not all intubations are done on board MERT. Sometimes, not often, medics got off the Chinook to collect their patient and couldn't get back on again. Chinooks were audible and visible from miles away, so there were times when, in between the 9-Liner and arrival, the landing site had stopped being a landing site and become a target. On a boiling August day in 2009 two medics with two soldiers from the Force Protection Squad jumped out of the back of the helicopter, knowing it would have to wheel away immediately, couldn't even wait the two minutes or so that it would have taken them to fetch the casualty back in. As they ran across the ground, the rotors kicked up a blizzard of dust and rocks, so they moved as fast as they could to the stricken patrol group, paying no heed to what might lie in the soil beneath them. As the helicopter moved away, it felt as if they had been abandoned on another planet in the glare of the sun and insanity of the terrain – a full-blown fire fight around them and, all the while, the patrol group searching for devices, marking them, calling out to the medics – what is technically known as a semi-permissive environment for doing emergency medicine. The casualty was a T1, in a bad way, lying between two vehicles for protection. He needed a surgical airway, but kneeling at his head would create a too solid, non-moving target, so instead the team leader lay as flat as he could by his patient's side on the hot, sandy ground and cut directly into his windpipe to create a space for a ventilation tube. Then he attached the tube to a portable manual resuscitator (not on MERT now, air from a plastic bag) and started to pump oxygen, squeezing the bag and finding enough quiet somehow amid the noise and haste to ensure a calm, regular rhythm, like a lung, in out, in out. And then twenty minutes that felt like twice that passed, and the rotors came back, thump thump, and the Chinook landed. Gathering the casualty up, running back, bagging him all the way, again not looking to see if the way was safe but this time getting back in and up and away.

Back on the helicopter, sometimes MERT had an audience in real time. There was room for those less badly injured, who'd walked up the ramp, shirtless and filthy, even if it meant they had to sit upright on an uncomfortable metal box full of medical supplies. Grey-faced from their own shock, they had nowhere else to look except at the sight of those others on the floor, hanging by threads, being fought for right in front of them.[5] All around, hanging from the red webbing across the walls of the cabin, were more blood products, and blood-stained gloves reaching for them, squeezing the bags in, pints and pints for humans who have lost more blood than they should have, and are only alive because they are young and battle-fit, and used to fighting, whatever the time and place. Monitors. Bips. Listen, try not to listen. Tangles of lines going in and out, not to be tripped over, not to be disrupted. Keep your arms in. Drilling, intubation, screaming, lines, tubes, monitors, bips. Watching, while others surround and save their mate.

Some of what the medics do looks really strange. Every single piece of information gathered during the Golden Hour is, well, golden. So in order not to forget it or waste time taking it repeatedly, MERT crew use Sharpies to write important data on whatever flesh remains undamaged on their patient – respiratory rates, heart rates – it's the best place of all for the next set of medics to find it, written on the body indelibly, in thick dark letters, signs of life. Writing on flesh, letters and numbers, where previously there had only been tattoos. Writing records was important, and not just those Sharpied on to patients. MERT crew tried to remember all their difficult cases, so they could learn from them. One team leader took his black plastic knee pads out just before each shift began and wrapped them in green sniper tape. Sniper tape is the military equivalent of duct tape – used for everything, and always a couple of rolls of it knocking about. It's fabric adhesive tape that tears off very easily and is flexible around odd shapes, and you can write on it. Inside the helicopter as the patient was stabilised or no longer needed his attention, the team leader straightened out his own leg and wrote on the knee pad, just the basics, to prod his memory when he was back in his quarters: time of treatment, levels of respon- siveness (E for Eyes, V for Verbal, M for motor), respiratory rate, heart rate, oxygen levels.[6] If the patient died, he crossed through the first line of information. When he got back, he entered the data in his own personal diary, with simple illustrations of stick men, showing where the wounds were and any other details he thought were important. Then he ripped the sniper tape off his knee pads and, because the adhesive is really good, stuck it on the diary page as well. It was an effective system, and it was adopted by the colleagues that came after him. When he got home, the diary was the basis for his research. Not a randomised control trial or anything formal: sniper tape from his knee pad. Research can take many forms. And taken together, all their tapes showed the statistical contours tightening – because of extreme resusci- tation techniques the chances of surviving severe injury between 2006 and 2014 went from 83 per cent to 92 per cent and holding.[7]

Ninety-two per cent: so still the 8 per cent chance, even if all the other odds are in their favour. The seated wounded learn in an instant that the hurly-burly of the cabin is better than the moment when the team leader sits back on their heels and reaches out to hold back the others with a gloved hand and speaks firmly but more quietly than before to call a halt. And they see suddenly that the pile of folded black plastic in the corner is in fact a pile of black body bags, and the crew moves as fast as possible to cover the dead. And then they watch as they go to whoever needs them next, past their failure, shifted a little way over. Later, one team leader remembered the sudden, intense loneliness he felt at the moment he called a death, as if he had been first to that point, after the casualty, and was waiting for everyone else to catch up, and that the seconds in which they did so, medic or comrade, were infinitely long. If life is difficult to measure in the back of a Chinook, then death can be even harder. Over the noise of the rotors medics can't hear breathing, can't feel a pulse, even though they check anyway. Sometimes the dust and debris covering a body are so thick, or the flesh is so burned, they can't get lines in, can't get monitors on. They can't do the tests they are supposed to do before calling a halt. Then sometimes they know, as soon as they look, that what is left on the floor cannot possibly be alive, even though it was loaded by the team medics as such, and they don't even begin, and instead one of them straight away reaches for the pile of black plastic.

And on they would fly, and then finally the helicopter would turn and bank to land at Bastion. Two landing pads. One, just outside the hospital, was named Nightingale (for what I hope is an obvious reason). And then, a short hop and the always impressive 180-degree turn to land at the dedicated helicopter landing strip, where the Chinooks lived all in a row, with MERT quarters just nearby. Even if it was due to go out again, which it often was, the pilots sat quietly for a few seconds while the giant rotors slowed down, and the engines ticked as they cooled and then finally apply a brake. They walk around the craft and check it for bullet holes and then finally sign it over to its ground crew engineers, who had waited, one ear permanently cocked since the arrival of the 9-Liner, which they also saw, until it returned safely (and they did all return safely). As the engineers refuelled it, MERT nurses cleaned the cabin clean of the blood on the thick rubberised lining on the floor. The Chinook's original fit had no blood mat, so fluids seeped into every crack and screw thread, and it was impossible to get clean or rust-free. The mat made everything easy, a big fluid spill kit wiped all manner of matter away, and while the nurses did that, they made a list of what supplies needed replenishing (everything usually) or what flew off during flight and needed re-fixing to the cabin walls. Bullet holes, nothing could be done about those, but they emptied the sharps bin and cleaned the windows and gathered up the blood-soaked dressings and never quite managed, no matter how hard they scrubbed, or how long the ramp was left open, to get rid of the smell of a ripped-open human being. There was not just blood to be cleaned away. Dust is more permanent than blood in Afghanistan. It has its own particular quality, very fine, and gets in everywhere, into the delicate electrics of monitors, engine parts, window frames. So afterwards ground crew cleaned as diligently as the nurses, a constant battle with blood and dust, while they waited for the next call, when they would all do it all again.

*

MERT service can come at a cost for those who work in the crews. Tinnitus is common – the ringing in the ears an unending echo of the shouting, chaotic soundscape of the Chinook cabin. Spines, backs, necks, shoulders, knees, all are affected by the weight bearing down on them shift after shift, and the constant vibration, leaving behind chronic pain and in some cases real, physical, career-ending disability. And these are just the things we know about now, only a few years after their final flight in Afghanistan in September 2014.

And there are other costs, yet to be quantified, of finding themselves in a place where they battled for survival every step of an uncharted way, and remember only competitions where they were not the master, and, where the handover was about failure, how they failed, where they went too far or not far enough and had to turn back alone, and where the pile of black body bags went down rather than gathering the dust circulating in the points of light shooting through the cabin where they worked. The anaesthetist who had intubated the patient on the ground between two vehicles under fire never knew what happened to him after he handed him over. A couple of months later he saw the man's parents on the television talking about their son who had died in Afghanistan, and he knew that his patient hadn't made it after all and he cried alone as he watched, as he cried when he told me about it, years afterwards. Six thousand five hundred cases transferred to Bastion by MERT, and most of their crew's personnel remember just one patient, usually one who ended the journey wrapped in one of the black plastic body bags.

But they know that if anyone can keep a life saved along the way, it is them, and the knowledge and the skill to do it never leave them. Almost everyone who served on MERT that I have ever met keeps a tourniquet in the glove compartment of their car, just in case. When it seems a lot to take in, all this business with blood and breath and extreme resuscitation, start there, in a glove compartment that probably looks like the one in most cars, with the car manual and the round tin of car sweets and the tourniquet, black strap and Velcro, that can stop a bleed, and save a life, wherever. Just in case.

*

And what of the soldiers on the ground who turn away in the grit sprayed by the Chinook's downdraught and then go back to their base, their vehicle, the war?[8] *Pay attention to what MERT leaves behind,* someone said to me in the course of my interviews. It was an excellent point. What happens to the people who saw their comrade fall, and to the medics who kept them alive until MERT thundered over? One CMT oversaw the loading of three very severely injured casualties after a day-long fire fight that had felt to him as if it had lasted ten minutes. They had driven to the landing zone, and he had been forced to put a line for fluids into a patient with half his head blown away, working in the back of the vehicle as it bumped along to meet the Chinook. He had been pretty chuffed by that, feeling like a real doctor, in gloves and stethoscope. It was night, pitch black, and the only light came from the unit's head torches until the back of the helicopter opened up and para-medics wearing night vision goggles moved forward to receive his patients. Not a second wasted, as was their way. The only contact he had with anyone outside the unit for weeks, and not a spare word spoken.[9] As the ramp closed up, a hand threw the yellow resupply bag out at him, as was also the way: swap a treated patient for the supplies used up, dressings, oxygen, fluids, IV lines. But he was distracted; now the patients had gone, he realised he had not had body armour on, had none on now and was at risk from enemy fire in the flashes of torch-light. He turned to begin thinking about where his armour was and, as he did so, a soldier from the unit, mistaking the yellow resupply bag for rubbish, picked it up and threw it skilfully back into the helicopter through the almost closed ramp gap.

Fury. The patients had needed almost all his supplies, and it meant he would be scrounging around for replacements until a new drop or a return to Bastion. The thought got him back to his vehicle, inside the door, too angry to sit down, standing at the back, holding on to the seat in front. Then, as they drove, he had time to gather his thoughts, to – as he put it – square himself away, and then for what he later thought was prob-ably twenty minutes he did nothing, as the adrenaline of the day drained from him. Then he began to shake, horrendously, unstoppably, before noticing his clothes were soaked in blood. Back at base he jumped out of the vehicle and stripped off his kit, to burn it until it was gone. Then he put on clean clothes. He remembered smoking ten cigarettes in a row, while drinking four cups of tea, without stopping.[10]

5

The Deal

BY THE TIME THE MERT helicopter bumps down on the Nightingale landing site outside the hospital in Camp Bastion, in
whatever remains of the Golden Hour, the deal with death
will be done. Lives will be dragged back from a point no one
had previously thought possible, escaping from the place that
is almost death, no looking back, one step, one pulse beat,
back into the light, life. But just like in the myths that are
scattered through human culture and history, where a deal to
cheat death always has consequences, it would appear that the
Golden Hour comes with a price.

We have known for some time that soldiers who have been
injured badly enough to lose limbs don't, in the words of my
head of department, do very well. Studies of amputees from
the Vietnam War show that after thirty years they experienced
multiple serious long-term health consequences. Those studies
have in turn generated projections of the cost of care for the
British amputee cohort created in Afghanistan (£300 million or
thereabouts, in case you are wondering). What all these studies
have in common is that they take the amputation as the central
feature of the casualty – that the problems somehow begin with
the amputation itself, and the consequences of living with fewer
limbs than nature intended. We are coming to understand that
thinking this way may not be enough. Amputation is part of, but
not entirely the cause, of the blighting of lives by severe casualty.

In 2002 a study was begun of American soldiers who had been severely injured in Iraq and Afghanistan. It went right back to the beginning of casualty, in careful measured steps. Severe injury could mean anything from musculo-skeletal damage (including, but not necessarily, amputation) to soft tissue disruption or organ damage. What all the injuries had in common was that the casualty required resuscitation in order to secure survival. The first phase of the study was concluded in 2014. It found that soldiers who had suffered and survived severe injuries were at greatly increased long-term risk of developing the significant chronic health conditions associated with old age: hypertension, diabetes, coronary artery disease and chronic kidney disease (just for starters – there are probably others). They could spot this only ten years after the earliest injuries had been sustained.

And there was more. This risk 'followed a dose response pattern': the more severe the injuries, the more complex the resuscitation, the greater the risk of developing these conditions earlier in life. Patients who survive severe injuries age faster than those less injured – depending on just how severe, it can be twice or even four times as fast.[1] So the science seems to be telling us clearly that the extraordinary techniques of resuscitation that we saw in the back of all those helicopters in the Golden Hour were not finite, but are instead negotiations to strike a deal for the life of the casualty. And the terms of the deal are becoming clear: life now; less life, and of poorer quality, later.

This is an early interpretation of the data, but it's thorough. The next phase, begun in 2016, looks at the possible reasons why (and quietly notes that this is all going to be so expensive).[2] The authors of the research paper have a hypothesis about the mechanism of this accelerated ageing. It goes straight back to those first moments of the deadly cascade, when the body does everything it can to hang on to the life draining out of it, all the different cellular mechanisms trying to compensate for the physiological abnormality. And one in particular: inflammation.

Inflammation is how the body responds to injury – a splinter in your finger, the cold virus, bacteria, avulsive amputations, all provoke the same fundamental response. The inflammatory mechanism is a chemical reaction: a range of different chemical cell types are sent to fight the injury wherever it is. They consume dead cells and work to expand blood vessels around the insult, to get more blood carrying more oxygen and therefore more energy to living cells in the area. They weaken cell walls to make them more permeable so blood can get to the area more quickly and start the healing process, which is why the splinter scratch or a paper cut in your finger gets red, swollen and tender, and why your nose runs when you have a cold to sluice out the virus.

Inflammation isn't self-limiting. The worse the injury, the stronger the inflammatory response. Scale up the swollen red scratch on your finger. Imagine how Mark Ormrod's inflammatory response reacted to his loss of three limbs, not to mention the burns and other trauma from the IED that blew him up into the sky. What happens in cases like Mark's has a name now: the inflammatory storm. Researchers looking into the genomics of inflammatory response to acute trauma reckon that up to 80 per cent of cellular pathways and functions are re-purposed in its early stages, during the Golden Hour.[3] So even as life is fought for and saved, at another level the storm rages on. Or, as a vascular surgeon once explained to me so that I would absolutely understand how serious this is, the inflammatory mechanism in acute trauma means global whole-body badness.

Global whole-body badness is worst of all in injured front-line soldiers. In Britain, until November 2016, front-line soldiers were all young, fit males. In the young, inflammatory systems are raring to go, ready to match up to anything, and so that is what they do, rushing, flooding out into a system already battered from the outside, and already weakened from the inside when the soldiers are thin and hungry, as they often were in front-line positions in Afghanistan – with no fat, no reserves, nothing in the way. It's different for girls. Female sex hormones make the inflammatory mechanisms operate more safely, protecting the female body from its hyperactivity. This may have something to do with the physical ordeal of childbirth: it depends on what kind of researcher is giving me the explanation.[4]

Eventually, when the bargain for life has been struck, when enough blood has been restored so that the lungs function again, and the pathophysiological shock has faded, the fluid that carried the inflammatory cells around the body begins to recede. In severe trauma it leaves behind debris in its wake, like those pictures of coastal towns and communities in Japan after the tsunami of 2011. Wreckage, toxic pollution, a body turned cannibal, full of acid, super-sensitive to further insults, especially bacterial, so very limited immune responses and much greater likelihood of sepsis (blood poisoning). Sepsis is the worst possible outcome for patients who are going to need a lot of surgery, because sepsis is a significant cause of post-operative death.

And the inflammatory storm never really goes entirely away. What may be left behind is a 'chronic pro-inflammatory state' – a mechanism that evolved to fix a human is itself broken, and its response is to overreact chaotically all the time. Look around at most of the complications experienced after severe injury: many of them may be due to the body being in this chronic pro-inflammatory state, working too hard and counterproductively to produce healing. So from whenever the analysis is done – three days after injury, six months into healing or a decade into living again – inflammation is likely to be at the heart of disappointing, painful, complex, expensive outcomes.

Or it might be something else, or inflammation in combination with an immune system suppressed by all that new blood being forced into it to maintain life at a more basic level. But whatever it turns out to be, this research, which looks at the specifics of severe injury and extreme resuscitation and sees them in terms of a whole life's impact, is the most important thing in this book. It is the scientists' answer to the hard question of what is going to happen. The work of the MERT allows us to see just how extraordinary extreme resuscitation is and how far we've come, but also to understand that it has consequences, this deal for life, and that it is often (but not always) only a beginning.

6

Field Hospital Camp Bastion (Bastion)

WELCOME TO BASTION, the hospital. If the arrival is by helicopter, to Nightingale, then the journey has been minutes from
the field, and the point of wounding and the shouting. Then
there is a bump down on the landing strip and the shortest of
journeys from there by ambulance to the receiving area, where
trauma teams wait in the sunshine, and then more rushing into
the trauma bay or operating theatre. But that's not how most
people arrived at the hospital at Camp Bastion.

Named after the high-strength concrete that was used in so
much of its construction, Camp Bastion was the biggest British
military installation since the Second World War. At its peak
it was the size of Reading, an entire town that appeared in the
desert, dense and sturdy, with ramparts and sentry posts and
then desert again, and some mobile phone masts marking the
world beyond. During 2008, after Mark Ormrod survived his
triple amputation and changed everything the medics understood about severe but survivable casualty, they turned what
had been a tented field hospital – brilliant but with limitations
– into a new hard-build facility, with the same full range of
life-saving infrastructure (scanning, communications, consultants) that could be found in twenty-first-century trauma units
at home. Extraordinary, but at the same time never a good

thing when a hospital at war moves from tents to solid structures. Bastion – throughout the rest of this book that name always means the field hospital at Camp Bastion.

Medics arrived at the camp in large military aircraft, C-17 Globemasters, long flights, uncomfortable, everyone in a middle seat in a bad economy class, but they long ago learned to sleep sitting up and where they could (most of them from being junior doctors in the UK during the 1980s). They sat, always just a few of them, scattered among hundreds of soldiers, some of whom would be their patients, but no one thought too much about that. Then, cabin lights suddenly went dark as the descent began and it all started to seem real. Darkness because higher altitudes were safe and the runway was safe, but the zone in between was not, and everyone, regardless of their experience, sensed the sudden vulnerability. When the lights went dim, and all that was left were the points of chemical green from luminous watch dials, body armour suddenly weighed heavy and no one recognised anyone else any more. All the same in tactical darkness, hiding the aircraft and hiding the hollow inside each of them, alone in the crowd, hemmed in by the stiff seat and the never-ending hum of the turbines. There were no other sounds from passengers, only from those charged with their safe delivery, who gave short orders about when to wait and when to move. Everyone felt every bump and jolt as the aircraft descended and their adrenalin spiked up and down.[1] Sudden decompression, a thump as the giant wheels went down, then the final bump of the landing. Then the wide-mouth ramp lowered and the passengers prepared to disembark.

The Afghan air is hot – 'like an oven', many people wrote in their diary. The night was cool, but the smell of a desert camp was the same whichever time and whichever desert, and so was the instant salt-lick of dust on their lips. For some it was utterly strange; for the experienced it was once again a sign that they were back in the Middle East. One surgeon arriving at Bastion in 2010 joined the others in walking down the ramp directly off the aircraft on to the landing strip. Looking around under a full moon and clear skies showed a distant, empty horizon. Meanwhile, as they marched away, he saw a dusty, worn-out, carbon copy of the long thick queue quietly facing in the opposite direction and waiting to board.

Everyone, including medics, had a briefing on arrival ('Why we are here'), and everyone, including medics, then went out to the range to test their weapons and their skills. But then they started to learn the standard things that new arrivals to war zones have always learned. What surrounds them, beyond the concrete of the camp, the landscape and beyond the air-conditioning and smell in the buildings, the weather. It was cold in the morning, and could be very beautiful: flat yellow desert bordered by dark brown mountains, sometimes hidden by dust clouds, sometimes lit orange by the sun, against the vivid blue of the sky. The cool clarity could be energising, making a first day at work something to relish. But by lunchtime it was very hot, especially under body armour, and they would be grateful the moment they pushed open the door of the hospital and walked into air-conditioning and stowed their protective shell. They learned to move at a clip across camp in daytime, to get back into the cool, except at night, which got cold quickly, a different shiver from that with air-conditioning. Evenings could be beautiful also, sitting back in a cheap folding deckchair outside their quarters, to look out on the geology, the eternity of space, night becoming dark, bounded by mountains that would be there long after the camp was taken down, sand blurring the traces until they were all gone.

They learned that the wind could get up strength in minutes, enough to gather up a desert full of sand and swirl it over the camp, blocking out the sun, covering everything, driving them into the nearest tent, provided it hadn't blown away. They would blink to clear the sand from their eyes until it stopped just as suddenly as it had started, and then they continued where they were going. Even when there wasn't a sandstorm, they learned that there was a technical term for the dust that settles on everything in their whole lives that wasn't in a hermetically sealed structure: dust and fines. Dust is dust wherever you go, but fines are particles smaller than dust that move in a mass like water and were dedicated to destroying their kit and were especially serious for MERT crews. Dust and fines are like nothing else, and everyone showed me film they had taken of them on their phones. Dust and fines, inches deep, like standing in shallow waves on a beach (or cocoa, said a practical one), washing over their desert boots, sinking them, centuries of it from a landscape worn fine by fighting and killing.

As they changed from military tunics to scrubs, they learned where there was a hospital laundry that turned around washing within a day, from the beds of casualties or backs of medics, and if they paid a little extra, the laundry ironed it for them. So they would really only need two sets of combats: one on clean, one in the wash. And if they didn't realise how MERT worked, they would once they understood about laundry. MERT always needed more, because in the very worst of times MERT was called out ten times a day, and they didn't change between flights, so the blood that went over the disposable aprons and gloves on to their combats stayed there for the whole shift.

*

For all the medics their first real day came when the watchmaster sent through the 9-Liner that also went out to MERT in their quarters. They learned a different kind of waiting in between signal and landing. The pulse quickened but not the pace, said one of the poets among them, and that readiness was all, both for themselves and for the place.[2] Drugs had to be stocked, in rows, trauma bays cleaned, sight lines straight and clear. There was an informal briefing, outlining what was expected, then everyone split into their teams. Trauma packs were taken out – pre-numbered, pre-printed labels for each patient, each T1, ready for them immediately, so there would be no waiting, no muddle with scans and labs when they were needed. Interpreters were called, if the 9-Liner indicated foreign nationals. The resuscitation trolleys were moved to one side of each bay so that the gurney carrying the casualty could fit in easily. The portable X-ray was positioned wherever the radiologist thought it should go, and the CT scanner was checked. (In the early days the vibrations of a helicopter landing nearby could set it off, so it had to be recalibrated carefully each time.) On the ward beds, heated mattresses were turned on because the rest of the place was cold from the air-conditioning. A runner arrived from the lab with shock packs for each bay expected to be in use. They contained red blood cells and fresh frozen plasma, and their boxes had a timer alarm that would ring if the contents were left for longer than thirty minutes. It was rare to hear the shock pack alarm because, no matter how much blood went in on MERT, more was always, always needed: at least one shock pack per amputation, so plenty were to hand.

But for now, there's time. Time for a brew, and a smoke outside the hospital, usually leaning against the same sunny outside wall where they took their breaks, listening out.[3] Then no more time. Dust swirled, and the helicopter approached the landing pad. Joggers from other parts of the camp, keeping fit by pounding the track of the Bastion boundary, stopped to watch, shielding their faces from the glare of the sun. Back inside, medics putting down their mugs, putting on their gloves and visors and bright green plastic disposable aprons.[4] Listening hard, and if they heard the helicopter bump down on the landing pad, they knew that life was not yet the master inside their cabin, and that their struggle would be at the limits of desperation.

Then the ambulances dashed forward the short distance. A look from the MERT crew inside told them if they needed to switch on their blue lights, to race to the hospital. Or that only a slower journey was necessary. Across a century, medics and nurses knew that look, that strain, dreading the work to come yet praying they needed to do it; anything the ambulance could unload alive was better than it creeping past them to the mortuary tent. Blue lights, speeding tyres through gravel, these things were at that moment, in the minds of the medics, who waited as medics have always waited, somehow a good thing.[5]

Stretchers were lifted out of the ambulance, and one of the MERT medics who had come in with the helicopter ran alongside with the stretcher crew, straight into the Emergency Department. At Bastion this was made up of six emergency trauma bays, marked by yellow lines, taped on the floor, and divider screens between each. As the casualty was wheeled into the bay, they gave a report and 'it is important that all receiving team members remain silent and listen', according to the textbook, so that everyone knew precisely what was required of them in what was left of the Golden Hour.[6] MERT had worked to keep the patient alive until this point, and now it was up to them to surround and save for the short journey between the trauma bays and the operating theatre. So more of what was done on MERT, done all over again (fresh dressings, fresh tourniquets), doing more of it (blood, fluids, analgesia). A bigger team than MERT. Here on the ground a trauma team leader, two nurses, two doctors, someone who did nothing but start and keep the records (with the biblical designation of 'scribe') for the patient, two airway specialists and a radiographer, who provided a detailed assessment of the casualty with images and scans (X-ray, ultrasound and CT). And there were other things to do, like rolling the patient carefully over to check their back (difficult to do on MERT, not enough room). And off they went, all at once. If all the bays were full, medics swarmed around their patients, filling the department; one of the deployed medical directors took to wearing a whistle on his lanyard in case control was lost in the room, but he never had to blow it.

It was not that different from what they would find in the trauma bay of a large NHS hospital, except the Bastion bays ran hot, with more patients in a week than most NHS trauma departments see in a year. Despite being a field hospital, in a desert, in the middle of a war, the Bastion Emergency Department ran better than most if not all NHS equivalents because, although it was small, it was perfectly formed and perfectly located. When the hard-build went up, they could make sure that the Emergency Department was within easy wheel of the ambulance bay, and that the imaging suite was directly next door, and the operating theatre also next door. And all of it actually next door, not down a corridor or round a tight corner that it was difficult to get stretchers down smoothly. This could be done in a hospital that was built from scratch and carefully planned, and really only does one thing (trauma), but not in the patchwork of nineteenth- and twentieth-century components that make up most of our current NHS provision.

And because Bastion medics didn't have to cope with long journeys to radiology and back, or wait for bloods, they could refine their system even further, by the smallest degrees. A small degree, a second gained in the Golden Hour, is part of the science of marginal gains. What had been two steps (resuscitation, then surgery) became one at Bastion because it could – resuscitation AND surgery AND imaging AND blood transfusions. Everything happening at once, every pulse beat fought for carefully planned and practised, full of expertise.[7] Be ready before they get into the bay. Move the patient once, from the stretcher to the operating trolley and use the move to check for injuries. Start at the top AND bottom of the patient. Get portable X-ray and ultrasound machines so they can work on the move, and get quickly out of the way, so the next person waiting can step into the space. At Bastion it was called Right Turn Resuscitation because it was a right turn into the Emergency Department, where the entire team was waiting. From a 360-degree battlefield to a 360-degree hospital, flying or on the ground, someone everywhere, working, surround and save.[8] Right Turn Resuscitation is fast and necessary for unexpected survivors, but it needs a whole team, and if it's instigated for patients who won't make it past the operating theatre door, then the team has been tied up when they could have been more use elsewhere. There's such a thing as 'over-triage', where things are imaged or intubated or done unnecessarily. And Right Turn Resuscitation is exciting and urgent, and teams can get carried away, which is why an experienced scribe is necessary so that, as each of them call out their activities for the record, control and pace are maintained. It needs a firm and experienced team leader for the same reason, and plenty of training in realistic rehearsal scenarios. But when it works, it works. Without it there would be far fewer unexpected survivors and no opportunity to learn the challenge of the scourge of Bastion, blast injury.

*

Surround and save and learn. This is what happens after the heartbeat under the soil has thumped and blown a human being up into the air with its force. Learning the consequences of an invisible wave, a 'blast wave', pulsing through a body, as damaging as the fragments that they can see and actually feel. It is difficult to overstate the power and consequences of the blast wave, so here is testimony from the first day of the battle of the Somme, 1 July 1916, as a young pilot from the Royal Flying Corps headed out over the La Boisselle salient. One of the huge shells that flew across the lines all day landed nearby:

> Suddenly the whole earth heaved, and up from the ground came what looked like two enormous cypress trees. It was the silhouettes of great, dark cone-shaped lifts of earth, up to three, four, five thousand feet. And we watched this, and then a moment later, we struck the repercussion wave of the blast and it flung us right the way backwards, over on one side.[9]

Or, as a scientist put it half a century ago: 'the Blast Wave is a shot without a bullet, a slash without a sword. It is present everywhere in its range.'

A blast wave is a pressure wave, and this scientist, Theodore Benzinger, had a decade that included the entire Second World War to study the effects of extreme pressure waves on human physiology. He became a leading expert, his insights and experiments so valuable that the American Air Force was prepared to overlook the fact that he was a Nazi, had worked with colleagues who used prisoners in their experiments, and had been one of the doctors on trial at Nuremberg. Benzinger's name had mysteriously disappeared off the list of defendants and he went back to work in his lab, before finally leaving Germany for good to work in the United States, where his eulogies noted not his Nazi past but the fact that he was the inventor of the ear thermometer.[10]

Blast is present – blast impacts – everywhere in its range. And from 2009 it was present in almost all the casualties who presented at Bastion. So learning blast was essential. Learning from every single blast injury casualty who passed through their hands, whether on the floor of the MERT helicopter or in one of the six trauma bays or the operating theatre at the hospital, where the surgeons and anaesthetists had a long time to get acquainted with the utter wreckage that was a human being, still smoking from the blast that brought them there. They learned not to be surprised when the body on the trolley was shorter than normal, because the feet, shins, thighs and sometimes pelvis were simply blown away and all that was left was in tatters, hanging limply over exposed bone, gaping holes through into the stomach, groin gone, yet somehow with oxygen circulating, life gripping on, a heart rate still fluttering in all the mess. Then they learned to find and accept the rest of it, everything blasted into their patient, in exchange for what was gone – pebbles and rocks, dust and debris, pieces of everyone else injured in the same blast, bones and flesh and skin suddenly mixed and indistinguishable. A piece of boot, a tough leather heel wedged between ribs. And the shrapnel of the bomb itself, whatever was to the bomb-maker's hand – nuts, bolts, ball-bearings, bicycle gear pieces, or grenade or mine fragments, twenty years in the rusting – dissolving in their sudden saturation of fresh, living blood.[11]

Not just bones and ligaments. The blast wave is especially dangerous to soft, air-filled organs. It bursts eardrums ('tympanic membranes' as they are known in the labs) – we used to think that it was the sound of the blast that did it, but now we know it's the pressure wave. Or the blast wave can perforate the gut, spreading infection from within, no help needed from external fragments. Only the human eye seems adapted to cope with the blast wave, because there is no air between its multiple fine layers. It helps if the eye is protected, which it usually was in Afghanistan by sunglasses, and if the eye's owner isn't looking at the blast when it goes off. So nothing much has changed since the Second World War here, although sometimes the place between the sinus and the eye socket, which does have air in it, can be affected and blown out through blast.[12] Lungs are also soft, air-filled organs. The lungs, with their finest of fine membranes, are the least dense organ in the entire body, made almost entirely of air.[13] Blast lung occurs when the force of the wave ruptures these finest of fine membranes, bleeding begins again, damage begins and by now you should know where this will end. Bad blast lung kills quickly, takes out the central mechanism to get oxygen in the blood, with blood coming back up the intubation tube as the lungs dissolve; there is nothing to be done. But blast lung can happen slowly, sneakily, and it's much worse in civilian victims of explosions, because they are usually injured in enclosed spaces (such as tube carriages), so the pressure on the fine lung membrane is more concentrated.[14] There are obvious things that can be spotted on a chest X-ray in the trauma unit and treated, but there are more subtle effects. A patient may present as 'not too bad' respiratory-wise, but within days their breathing has become laboured, they've got chest pain and their now permanent cough has blood or foam in it.[15] If caught in time, blast lung can be treated with oxygen therapy, via a face mask or a ventilator, and slowly the membrane recovers and strengthens and can begin to work again.

7

Mark Ormrod (2)

LEARNING, AND SO MUCH OF IT LEARNED from the first surviving triple amputee who was rushed into their operating
theatre on Christmas Day 2007. Everyone who had seen what
remained of Mark in the bomb crater assumed he had died
en route to Bastion. The leader of the MERT team who collected him assumed he was dead – there was no discernible
pulse or circulation that could be felt above the vibration of the
aircraft, and anyway no one had ever survived those kinds of
injury before. During the checks prior to declaration of death,
the medic noticed Mark's eyeball flicker. Not dead after all.
Mark received three pints of replacement fluid via his hip bone
and, by the time the helicopter landed at Bastion, was revived
enough to talk. Nonsense mostly, but actual talking. The rest
of his unit spent the day (Christmas Day) sharing a roast beef
dinner at the base, and were able to enjoy it, even those still carrying the singes and grazes from being near the blast, knowing
he had made it out of the helicopter alive, and that someone
had thought to tell them.

Inside the theatre Mark was surrounded by an entire
team of surgical consultants, a neurosurgeon, an orthopaedic
surgeon and a general surgeon. For as long as he could hold
out they worked, and it took twenty-four pints of blood to keep
him with them throughout. They took off his tourniquets and
then the remnants of his right leg. His left leg was amputated

through the knee, and all the delicate machinery that runs through the knee – muscles, hamstrings, tendons, ligaments, all coming together in a small, crowded space – everything was cut and tidied back, along with the veins and nerves and soft tissues. The bone ends were filed to remove any sharp edges, and muscles brought down to create a flap which in turn created his stumps.

So on they worked. Mark's right arm was destroyed; there was no chance of piecing it back together. Instead the struggle was to amputate as low down as possible, leaving as much healthy tissue beneath the shoulder as could be managed. Shoulders are needed for body shape, for holding up clothes, for balance, so surgeons never cut into a shoulder if they can conceivably help it. His left hand had been split by the piece of shrapnel, from the palm under the index finger to the little finger – unbandaged, there was a hole that Mark could look through – but it was salvageable, so they worked on it, with extraordinary care, knowing the stakes, and then wrapping their work to protect it in so many layers of bandage that it looked like a white boxing glove.

On they worked to remove the debris strewn by the blast throughout what was left of Mark's body, excising, washing, debriding – the surgical removal of dead or dying tissue so that wound healing can begin. War means many things, but above all it means surgeons standing for hours debriding, piece by piece, with gravel clattering into metal trays, again and again, gently syringing wounds clean, until the grey is gone and only healthy pink remains. They removed the haemostatic dressings, clumps of them buried deep, tossed on to the floor of theatre, to clear up later. They closed up the broken major blood vessels and cauterised the smaller ones. Mark had a series of deep, teardrop-shaped burns on the left side of his back which needed cleaning and treating. Later he would ask if they had damaged the huge and elaborate tattoo he had there (they hadn't). Towards the end his new limb ends were packed in gauze bandages and the wounds dressed. Then it was the

Critical Care ward, until he could go home, still punctured with lines pumping in clotting agents, blood products, fluids, antibiotics. His own personal legion of Critical Care nurses never leaving his side. Still alive, the first triple, but within weeks more joined him, so that, although his journey would be long, at least he would no longer be alone.

8

Bastion's Medics

AS THEY LEARNED THEIR WORK at the hospital, so the medics learned about each other. As in life, in books. So, meet the junior trauma surgeon. You might meet him anyway, in an NHS unit, if you need a surgeon to look at a hand or hip or leg that has been badly damaged. You'd never know that he's been in Iraq, and that while he was there he counted the mortars that fell around him while he was in the operating theatre (forty-six), and that one night he lay flat on his belt buckle (military terminology for lying down as low as you can because people are firing at you) waiting to treat a casualty while a fire fight raged directly over his head. Or that he's been in Afghanistan, and if there are more wars somewhere else, then he'll go there. Which is why I can't tell you his name, but I can tell you that when he does cardiac resuscitation he whispers the song 'Nelly the Elephant' to help him keep time, beating down hard and rhythmically, as the elephant SAID goodbye to the CIRCus, keeping a heart beating for the length of a song and several choruses until it could run on its own, picking up the rhythm, flipping back and forth to life. He does that today, and he did it in the trauma bays of Bastion, and that was how his colleagues got to know him.

The worst day the junior trauma surgeon ever had in Afghanistan started with a repatriation ceremony. He had woken up, put on his uniform and stood to attention in the open square at Camp Bastion as the coffin of a soldier who had been killed in the field was carried on to a Globemaster transport plane. Absolute silence, except for the voice of the chaplain and then the Last Post, and always, somewhere in the background, the Afghan wind in the desert. Then he had gone slowly and quietly to the hospital for his shift. No patients, just paperwork, left to his own devices and thoughts, never particularly welcome after a repat. But at 5 p.m. something worse happened. A 9-Liner: four serious casualties, two of them very bad indeed, and they'd waited for thirty minutes before it was safe for MERT to land and collect them.

Too long. With one already dead, MERT crew turned away to work on the other, still very bad when unloaded. Right turn at Bastion, everyone there pushing forward to surround where he lay, no heartbeat, so the junior surgeon opened his chest, and reached in for the heart itself, massaging it hand to heart, no ribs or chest in between, no muttered song for rhythm, just thin sterile gloves gleaming with blood on a pair of hands and the muscle itself, lying between them, not moving, not responding. Keep going. Blood and adrenalin in through the lines to help him, and finally, after four minutes the surgeon felt a flutter between his hands, and then a twist and then a rhythm, and then he could actually see it moving in the middle of all that blood, beating on, and then – not that he needed it – the monitor bipped a confirmation. No more time to listen, as there were many more injuries, but now the veins that held the lines were shutting down, so blood must be leaking out somewhere, blood pressure falling, patient falling back, so the team went back after him. His leg was gone, so an amputation to remove what remained just below the knee was being done. Lacerations to the lung, but not serious. Where else? Open up the stomach – blood so dark and deep – a huge haemorrhage, still bleeding, unstoppable, but they tried, more blood in the lines, back and forth, heart massage, but this time no fluttering, no movement, and the team leader called a halt.

Different work at the end of a life. Sewing up the wounds made by the blast and those others they had made fighting for survival. The work of an hour or more always, and dreaded, but he sewed slowly and carefully, the repat ceremony coming back to him with every suture and clip, because he knew that now there would be another. More remembering: the last time he had done this for a young dead soldier, a year earlier, another tour, Iraq. An open chest, blood pouring on to his shoes and the drapes around the trauma bay, litre after litre, and then the team leader said that he needed to think about stopping, and then that he should stop. And even now a year later, when he knew nothing could be done, it was the same despair, wishing with all his heart that something had been possible, that they had kept going out and kept hold of him somehow until they could see the way back.

Four casualties came in. One dead on arrival, one dead in the trauma bay. And the day that was now a night went on. A morgue team arrived to collect his patient, and he pulled off his blood-soaked gown and gloves. The other two casualties were out of the trauma bays now, their lives secured in place, but they needed surgery on their injuries. So he had an hour to rescrub, put on fresh gown and gloves and then go back in – this time a hand to be saved. He remembered very little of the details. Sleep at 2 a.m. and then back into theatre first thing, and bed again the next 2 a.m., and theatre first thing for the next three days. As he operated, MERT landed and unloaded and went out again, and the procession of trolleys before him never stopped: gunshot wound to the stomach, fragmentation wounds to the face, blast injury to the lung, amputating one leg, amputating both legs, hand trauma, fragmentation to the upper arms, twenty of them, and then again the take-backs and the reworkings and the ward rounds. Exhaustion, drifting off during the moments of break – understanding what a thousand-yard stare was because he had one. Finally sleep. And then the next morning, beret on, stand upright, repatriation ceremony for the first death, in howling wind and then driving rain and constant flashbacks to the operating theatre and the moment the halt was called. The storm raged outside all night, but he slept through it, and the next morning the air was clear and the mountains to the north beautiful in the sunlight, and he could see all their features, rivers and ridges, where the sand of the desert met the warmth of the rocks at its edge. Closer, somewhere in the camp, small birds playing in the sand, two days of quiet to follow.[1]

Except that he'd adjusted his definition of quiet. Quiet could still mean days and days of ward rounds, and take-backs and trimming and re-trimming of stumps, because the blast wave still needed resisting days after it had exploded. Blast injury wasn't new for him. He'd been in Iraq, when blast casualty from IEDs was an 'emerging injury pattern', something to be written about in short articles, rushed to medical journals, to let everyone who would come next know that this new weapon was causing significant injury patterns and casualty numbers, a complex of casualty 'often resulting in traumatic amputation'.[2] In 1914 surgeons had written home of the mutilating wounds of modern warfare, where 'the amount to be done in a short time is large, and much increased by the multiplicity of wounds', and that they already somehow understood 'many surprises must be expected both in the direction of recovering and of final failure.'[3] The same thing, across a century. The junior trauma surgeon thought about that when he did a last check on his patients before going off duty. In the low night light of the Bastion hospital ward he could see every bed used, but not full, every leg and some arms gone into a yellow bag. He stood at the door and felt connected to all the military surgeons who had gone before him, standing in dimly lit places and seeing in hospital the lives saved, blighted and failing there all at once, surgeons who had gone back to their tents and hurriedly written up a warning and sent it off, or a diary to seek sense in the madness. And then he turned and walked back to his tent.

Meet some more of the others. Meet the plastic surgeon. He was the first plastic surgeon to come to Bastion, and he came as part of the general trauma team, before anyone real-ised that it would be the plastics lot who stayed behind at the operating tables, hour after hour, even though this happens every time medics go to war. Even in 1914 a surgeon had written home warning those that were embarking for France that 'skin-grafting and other plastic operations will have to be extensively practised'.[4] When he looked back, the plastic surgeon didn't remember any days in particular, just reckon-ings he'd made while standing at an operating theatre table, alongside unexpected survivors. Plastic surgeons learned to read the wreckage of the human beings brought to them like no one else. Orthopaedic surgeons focused on the bones that were their responsibility. Everything else, all the rags and sanded shreds, where veins and nerves end, what comes out from under the tourniquet when it's finally safe to loosen, that was down to the plastic surgeon.[5] If they weren't careful, wreckage became war-like scrap – an official term, by the way, for military rubbish, to be disposed of. To stop that disintegra-tion, bleep the plastic surgeon and watch him be careful at the operating table, for as long as the patient's own physiology will let him, fingertip searching the debris for the material blasted deep into the body's layers, debriding putrid flesh back to some-thing pink and healthy, putting it back together wherever he can. Trimming tissue, muscles, nerves, refining the new edges of body at the stumps.[6] Plastic surgeons: the men and women who can deal with soft tissues, the nerves, veins, arteries, bits and pieces, fingers, scalps, ears, lips, the really small things, reconstructing the human part of human beings.[7]

The plastic surgeon also learned that soldiers never listen, no matter how much he told them to keep their gloves on and not to cut the fingers off, because if they did that, the more likely it was that he would have to cut their fingers off – that little layer of scientifically designed fabric does do what it is supposed to do. But Spitfire and Hurricane pilots wouldn't wear their gloves or goggles in the Battle of Britain for the same reasons: it was hot, and they worried that gloved hands were less sensitive or quick on their instruments and weapons. So sixty years apart both of them lost fingers and eyelids and flesh when it could have been saved, but who's to argue with the young man with his finger on the trigger or the bomb detector as he goes forward into the fire.

The plastic surgeon has deployed eight separate times to war zones and, as I write this, he's training to deploy again, not to a war this time, but to what is left behind by civil war, to train surgeons how to rebuild humans in an 'austere environment', even when that austere environment is the place they call home. I can't tell you his name either, or the name of the place he will be posted to when this book is published. But I'll ask him to tell me about it when he comes back, whatever he can, because he's got an eye for detail, like most plastic surgeons. He saw Bastion when it was just an air base, and right outside its relatively puny fences were the adversaries, looking back at him and sometimes firing rockets. Bastion had a tented hospital, like all field hospitals before it, but one that grew and grew, day by day, wings and wards added like a game of dominoes spreading out as the camp itself turned from an air base in 2003 into a fortified settlement into a city, secured by guard posts and blast walls, made of Bastion concrete: miles and miles of them, no more worrying what was beyond the wire. Camp Bastion, like all modern cities, turned into a giant car park as more and better military vehicles appeared in longer and longer rows, in their identical beige-grey desert camouflage paint coat. And in 2008 the plastic surgeon saw the hard-build hospital go up: huge pieces unloaded from the back of transport aircraft and bolted together. First one storey and then a second, and a whole spiral staircase clamped up the side from one to the other. A tarmac entry for ambulances, reinforced floors to take the weight of the new scanners, which he was happy to see because they in turn took some of the weight off him, telling him where the fragments were and where they were not, so he didn't have to waste time and his patient's blood searching for them.

Even when the hard-build was finished, they kept the old tented field hospital just in case the new one was overwhelmed. There's a technical term for when that happens: Going Black. Going Black would have been catastrophic – military operations would have been suspended until the hospital could readmit casualties. Troops would have struggled to maintain morale, knowing the hospital was failing and there was nowhere for them to go when they fell.[8] But there was always somewhere, and the need was never so great that every single medic in the camp was mobilised at once; throughout the war teams gathered on their shift and stayed away when they needed rest.[9] The tented field hospital was also there in case the new hard-build came under attack. Anyone who had been in Iraq knew how it felt to operate with mortars falling all around, but at Bastion the blast walls held fast and the perimeter grew beyond the range of all but the occasional mortar or rocket going off somewhere in the distance.

But an attack was constantly in the mind of the Bastion Deployed Medical Director. Always a consultant, preferably in an acute specialty, the Deployed Medical Director had the last word on things like the boundaries of resuscitation (who was treated and for how long, and how many resources were used on them). They made sure that good ideas like Right Turn Resuscitation were implemented. They managed highly intense staff in a high-intensity environment. They thought about hard and difficult things all day, and this was particularly the case for the Deployed Medical Director in 2009, because he knew exactly what a hospital looked like when it was part of the aftermath of an attack.[10] He had been in Belfast in 1991, when a bomb exploded in the fire exit tunnel serving the basement social club of the military wing of the Musgrave Park Hospital. The social club was full because the rugby World Cup final was on, and many of the medics were watching it on the big social club television. The explosion collapsed the two floors above into the basement, trapping the wounded and destroying the accident department, resuscitation room and operating theatre. Two medical staff were killed and nine others badly injured, including two child patients in the newly opened paediatric orthopaedics ward.

Preparations for an attack had been made which assumed that the accident department would be available, but it was not, and everything that would have been needed was destroyed along with it. Resus facilities were improvised in the road near the building by the anaesthetist, who scavenged drugs and equipment from Critical Care. There were no hi-vis jackets or protective clothing, no pre-planned system of radio communication and no triage labels of any kind, so patients went off in ambulances to other hospitals with staff having to remember what they had been told. No one knew if a second attack would happen at any minute. So in addition to a Major Accident Plan they needed special incident boxes, protective clothing and documentation prepared and ready for use in a pre-designated alternative treatment facility somewhere else on their grounds. After Musgrave Park he switched specialties to emergency medicine, and Musgrave Park was always some-where at the back of the Deployed Medical Director's mind, ticking over, causing him to refine and reshape the smallest detail so that a disrupted hospital could go on functioning. So the field hospital tent stayed, and got a name – Resilience – even though it was only used once, when the CT scanner was being installed in the hard-build and everyone had to be moved out back to the tents to let the technicians work.

A 9-Liner and then the sound of 'Doe, a Deer, a Female Deer' beeping from his pager called the hand surgeon to the trauma theatre at Bastion. (As part of the plastic surgery cadre, he was on call all the time, and he had the tune of 'Do Re Mi' from *The Sound of Music* as his bleep, not because he liked it but because he hated it, so he always took notice when it played, like hearing fingernails on a blackboard.) Like the others, he waited behind a yellow line until the anaesthetist called him forward, and although there may have been burns to the face or body that required his skills, the cases he most remembers, that he cannot quite yet live with, are those that involved hands.

Hands are about living, holding, doing the smallest thing, feeling the softest touches, fingertips. Hand surgeons work close up, their visual field no longer than the middle finger of their patient, turning the hand over and back, thinking, mending, saving. Hand surgeons are determined and clear in their mission: that they will never amputate hands that might be saved. The hand surgeon brought this certainty to Bastion, brought it every day he walked into theatre, and began to understand that military casualty only strengthened that resolve. As his colleagues worked on patients who had lost both legs, he knew how important it would be to their recovery that they had their hands. Every bit of function he could save, no matter how small, would enable their journey through their new lives. A new determination and resolve: they need their hands if they lose their legs.

'Doe, a Deer', a very bad day, called to theatre past a full set of trauma bays working on very severely injured casualties, and with five dead outside waiting for transport to the mortuary. His patient: both legs gone at thigh level, a mangled left hand and a right hand intact, although the elbow was smashed through with shrapnel. The hand surgeon was called forward to the left hand, cleaned up and lying waiting for him on the table. It was staying on, and he was going to fix it, on this very bad day, no matter what. The pieces he could see were pieces that could be mended and made back into something that worked and even looked like a hand. And so he did, disappearing into his own world as around him the surgeons and anaesthetists heaved stumps closed, and pumped in fluids and dragged life forward, one pulse beat at a time. He worked on, and the pieces came back together, more work to be done later, but good for now. Then the elbow – not much to be done there, so the right arm would never flex properly, but there were two hands still, to grip the equipment in the rehab unit, to offer in a handshake, to begin to feel a way forward in the new world he had come to inhabit. Throughout the very bad day those two hands at the end of two arms kept the hand surgeon going. No compromise, work done, as promised. Resolve strengthened.

A week later. Another patient, both legs removed above the knee, almost as bad as it got, and the blast wave had also blown open the right hand – both arteries in the wrist blown away and open fractures in the palm. He'd done the one the week before, and this one didn't look much worse so he'd save this one too, and make rehab a little easier. The work: restoring the veins and arteries, making decisions about shunts or grafting, about how to tidy up the wrist that pumped in the blood, and sensation and function. Painstaking work, time-consuming work: at least half an hour to start with, bent in close, his own gloved fingers touching and testing those he could save, fifteen minutes gone. Tunnel vision, save the hand, I can save the hand. Then 'Stop', someone said firmly, at the borderline of saying and shouting. He looked up. The rest of the team had stopped, and they were all looking at him. There was more than a right hand on the table, there was an entire body, and it was still bleeding what little remained of the whole body's blood out through the smashed arteries at the wrist. The voice again, the team leader, ordering him to amputate the hand immediately or the patient would die: not a risk but an absolute certainty of death. He performed the amputation quickly, neatly (though he always describes it as 'chopping'). Technical term: fixation error – fixation on the hand and his ability to save it, hearing only his own resolution, losing the sense of the whole life.[11] And then he stepped back from the table to allow another trauma surgeon his space.

*

Some of the most difficult decisions taken by the Deployed Medical Director related to local patients, Afghans civilians, their families and others. Locals made up the majority (probably as much as 80 per cent) of the patients cared for during the lifetime of the hospital. During the war there were no Afghan hospitals with the technology or capability to ventilate patients with severe chest wounds, therefore leaving Bastion meant death. So anyone intubated who could not be returned to Britain had to stay at Bastion until they could breathe unaided, which sometimes took days or weeks. They were discharged only when it was certain they could survive away from Bastion: probably in a local hospital that was under severe stress, and which could only provide medical care for two or three hours a day, where the rest of the time they would be looked after by their families. So beds remained occupied by those who were not badly injured British service personnel, and sometimes there were no spare beds. Meanwhile no one knew when the next 9-Liner would come in and everything the hospital had would be needed for some of their own. To paraphrase one of the earliest deployed medical directors, an extended field hospital stay provided a combination of quality assurance and professional insurance (surgeons could be sure their work had worked), yet it threatened to undermine the field hospital's core objective: to support the military effort.[12]

On some days, though, that decision wasn't very hard at all, such as the evening when five Afghan National Army soldiers came in, all in one go, packed into one Chinook. All T1s, the very worst, listed on the whiteboard in the trauma bay area:

Trauma Bay 1	Head trauma, bleeding from carotid. Airway obstruction.
Trauma Bay 2	Sucking chest wound + cranial laceration. Shallow breathing. Weak pulse.
Trauma Bay 3	Shrapnel left arm, chest, both eyes. Massive head laceration, brain exposed.
Trauma Bay 4	Shrapnel wounds, concussion, in and out of consciousness.
Trauma Bay 6	Shrapnel, arm + left eye gone, facial laceration.[13]

And so they were taken back and forth to theatre, over and

over, because there was the time and the need to do really complex reconstructions that were all the patient was likely to get. So a huge workload for the plastic surgeons, rebuilding faces, eyelids, arms, hands, bodies. There was no surgical microscope at Bastion – microsurgery was done back in the UK, at Birmingham – so they couldn't fix the really fine intricate structures that needed microscopes and precision instrumentation, as they would do at home. So they used the techniques demanded by the injuries of other, older wars, where equipment was less sophisticated but the damage the same. In 1940 the plastic surgeon Archibald McIndoe was confronted with another set of unexpected survivors: RAF aircrew, their faces and hands burned away in exploding Spitfires, Hurricanes and Lancasters. He needed to restore whole noses, chins, cheeks, not with small grafts but big, one-off reconstructions. So he used the technique of tube pedicles, a procedure in which whole sections of skin are raised on three sides but keeping their blood supply connected on the fourth. Their open end is moved up to where skin was damaged or gone, gradually, stage by stage – 'waltzed' up a limb – stitched in place, from a shoulder to the face for instance, or a thigh to an arm. Then, when the blood supply had reconnected, it was snipped away from their original site and sewn up to make a whole new cheek or chin or lip, all in one go. No need for microsurgery, but the patient mustn't move their arm or shoulder where the graft came from until the surgeon said they could. No one does this now, because it takes so long and because they have microsurgery, but pedicles work and stay fixed, and at Bastion, with local patients, they had time. Military medics have to know a century's worth of medical techniques, because they never know what they will be called on to do, under what circumstances. Something to think about for a new generation of surgeons who don't do old-school procedures.

Perhaps the hardest part would have been explaining to a patient that they couldn't move their arm for the next week if surgeons didn't speak Dari or Pashtun or any one of ten other languages common in Helmand (there are thirty or more across the whole country). But fortunately they didn't have to, because of what were always known as the Terps. Interpreters were crucial to the functioning of the wards at Bastion. Many of them had some medical experience, had been nurses or orderlies in Afghan city hospitals, and once they got used to the wounds and their treatment, medics only had to start off with a full sentence or two and the interpreters nodded and gave a full set of instructions to the patient. They came without fear to the bedside of children, and Afghan soldiers and CPERS (Captured Personnel on Operations). There was an interpreter there for every extubation of an Afghan – the opposite of intubation, the removal of breathing tubes – who explained what was happening and asked the patient to cough and then quickly translated as the situation was being explained by the various consultants and nurses, the eyes of the patient flicking anxiously back and forth from the speaker of the language they knew to the faces of the men and women who stood in authority. They advised the medics on religious and cultural issues, such as diet and when and how the beards of the unconscious devout might be shaved. They stayed in their Terp roles for years, and medics who deployed several times to Bastion were always pleased to see them again in their wards, as if they had been waiting for them to come back.

When you think of the hospital at Bastion, make sure you have room in your mind for the Terps, because they were always there, and the hospital couldn't have functioned without them. They lived in their own tents, close to the hospital, and they often invited the medics back for talks and tea and a little light jewellery trading. Mining probably began in Afghanistan thousands of years ago, and there were still tourmaline, rubies, emerald and lapis lazuli to be bought and taken home for presents, although the plastic surgeon is equally proud of the cufflinks he had made in one of the engineering tents at Bastion out of used brass cartridge rounds.

And they are the only group that I have not been able to

reach for this book. Most interpreters have tried to slip back into their lives in Afghanistan without anyone noticing at the end of the war. Only those working in front-line posts between 2012 and 2014 have been allowed entry into the UK, and, as far as any of us can tell, that category did not include those working at the hospital. Afghanistan's own hospitals need them to work there, but it would mean exposing the kinds of expertise they could only have gained at Bastion, and that is a death sentence. The medics who came home worry about them constantly, try to find them, to make contact, to bring them here, but none of them has so far been successful. They all had the same expression when I mentioned Terps – regret, worry, fondness, resolution – and as soon as they'd finished talking to me went back on email, pressing the cause of the men they left behind. It's perhaps worth saying again: most of the patients in Bastion were Afghans, needing weeks and weeks of work, and this would have been impossible without the Terps.

Among the Afghan patients were not just army, police and civilians but also CPERS, although most just called them 'enemy combatants' (and in other parts of the camp they called them 'detainees', but never ever 'PoWs'). They all had a call on the medical facilities at Bastion, and the principles used to treat them were the same no matter what. Save, maintain survival, strengthen, reconstruct. Keep alive, no matter who or what. Then, when they could survive, they were collected and taken somewhere else, to another hospital or to an internment facility.[14] So there was a double pressure to move these particular patients out of the wards, to free up beds and to begin inter-rogation for intelligence that might include information that would prevent future casualties being created that would need those beds. Meetings ran long over schedule and past politeness as surgeons and clinicians argued about who could and should be moved out of the hospital wards. Daily reckonings, never getting any easier as the war went on.

Like the time a Chinook pilot who flew his MERT team out to casualties every day was called out to take an Afghan baby, dangerously ill with meningitis, from a local town to a civilian Afghan hospital. He had a new baby at home and, like all new parents, was suddenly super-sensitive about the infection. The Afghan child would almost certainly die without access to the antibiotic therapies only held at Bastion. So he ignored the MERT team leader, ignored the watchmaster, ignored the air traffic control tower at the Bastion airfield who tried to make him turn round and bumped down at Nightingale to deliver the child there. He'd flown mission after mission, in the heaviest of fire – had walked round his Chinook night after night to check it for bullet holes – but the child was suddenly his patient, the only one he would ever have, so worth the consequences, worth the loss of the bed. He never found out what happened to her, but he knew for certain that, if the decision fell to him again, it would go the same way.[15]

One day in January 2010 four beds were in use in the Bastion operating theatre at the same time, drawing on all the available skills in the place. It was a 'Mass Cas' – a mass casualty event – not of the same vehicle or unit, but of the same family. An entire Afghan family, injured by an IED, treated at an American unit in the field and then sent to Bastion once they were stable. The youngest, a baby, had died of head injuries soon after wounding, and a ten-year-old had suffered dreadful abdominal injuries. An American surgeon, posted to Bastion to support an ongoing offensive, found himself leading the teams treating the family, and in particular the badly injured child. There was a reason he had not gone into paediatrics, he remembered: because the pain of losing children despite his work and expertise was unbearable. And children die so easily, so quickly, when he thought he'd saved them, maintaining their blood pressure until the very last moment, and then they race their pulse up high and simultaneously lose their blood pressure down low – they crash hard – and then they die.

After five days of treatment most of the family had recovered and were ready for discharge. Only the ten-year-old in ITU ward bed number 7 remained. She had survived four separate surgeries to repair her intestines and abdominal wall, but her first tentative steps on the path to survival were dogged by sepsis. Sometimes her kidneys worked, sometimes not. Sometimes her white blood cell count was almost zero, other times almost normal. Hour by hour surgeons and nurses sat by her bed, wondering what else they could do, with interpreters coming and going, no one far from despair. Like the adults usually in the beds, she struggled in the nightmare world of sedation and pain, twisting in the bed, pulling at her lines. The surgeon decided to lighten her sedation very carefully, moment by moment, so that she could hear her father leaning over her and repeating low and gently, in Pashtun, that she should try not to pull at the tube in her throat, or the so many lines connecting her little body to the machines and fluid bags that kept her alive. She was just conscious enough to hear him, to understand and to nod her head obediently to her father.

Ten days later the child was recovering. One by one her problems were fixed, and her throat tube was removed and the lines replaced by food and drink. She sat up in bed, she could walk as far as her father in the chair, and was strong enough to climb into his lap. And one day her father came and she got up, and together they went home. The surgeon remembered all his patients, but he remembered the children the best. Afghan families were huge – a family of nine after the family of five – even though he never knew their names or enough of their language to talk to them. So many children, always at Bastion. One British medic sent home for an acute paediatric textbook because he simply didn't have the experience demanded by their casualty. He brought it home, battered and stained, pages falling out because he had used it every single day of his deployment.

*

But somehow they learned, just as surgeons had learned in other wars. They learned that, no matter how good the kitchen food was, it got boring (and it was better if they didn't think too hard about the roasting tins, which were sometimes borrowed by the trauma teams to catch the blood from patients as it poured off the operating table), so food parcels, the great staple of morale in the British Army, found their way to Bastion in the twenty-first century just as they had to the Western Front a hundred years before. The plastic surgeon liked cheese in his, preferably cheddar because it lasted longer, but anything with really strong flavours worked, such as smoked and tinned fish. If you've ever wondered who actually eats smoked oysters in a tin, the plastic surgeon is one of them, but only when he is on deployment.

If they wanted a walk that felt a little like a walk did at home, they could go and ask to borrow the sniffer dogs and take them out, on leads. The creatures seemed to enjoy Camp Bastion more than anyone, but then dogs enjoy almost anywhere. An emergency physician, Bastion's own Kipling, who wrote poems as well as diaries, wrote about them and the group of volunteers who gathered outside the working dogs pound every evening:

> *There are two types of dog and they differ –*
> *There is one type you don't want to stroke –*
> *The Labs and the Spaniels are sniffers,*
> *The Alsatians will go for your throat.*[16]

There were dogs in the pound that the doctors recognised because they had also been flown into Bastion injured. The vet had to be called to treat them, and sometimes this took a little time (no room on the 9-Liner for non-humans). One of the busiest MERT flights ever involved nine casualties, most walking, and a sniffer dog who had spent too much time searching for explosives and collapsed from heatstroke. Back in the trauma bay at Bastion they badly wanted to run lines into him to restore his fluids, but they resisted and waited for the vet.

On his first tour the plastic surgeon made a volleyball

court, scrounging gravel to mark out the lines and sewing a net for games in the late evening in the last of the light, when the hospital was quiet. He was really pleased when he went back for his last tour to see that it was still there, and people still found it useful at the ends of their Bastion day to split into teams and remember who was looking after the ball, and laugh and run their way into sundown. On the last tour he noticed that the blast walls now completely encircled the camp, even the long runway, and that the flags were almost permanently flying at half-mast. They hardly ever used the tannoys, because there were simply too many times when the news was too bad; instead, messages about deaths were carried to the various parts of the camp in person, and everyone obeyed the protocols quickly because they'd had a lot of practice. And he decided to make something at Bastion that wouldn't die or fly away or turn into a scar or stump, just for himself, so he built a garden.

He marked the garden out with wooden fencing scrounged from somewhere, and wedged terracotta pots into the dust and filled them with strong little plants and arranged them all in a neat, elegant scheme. Salads, herbs and plants whose names he never discovered but which grew and grew despite the heat and desert. There's even a technical term for them now because there have been hundreds of these defiant gardens – built in worlds surrounded by war and violence, offering sustenance, refuge, testimony, relief. He thinks of it now as just a little patch, but scale isn't important. With defiant gardens, even a micro-restorative environment is restorative, in an unexpected multiplicity of ways.[17] There were many gardens built at Bastion, but they could only really be appreciated from a helicopter in daylight, and usually people in helicopters in daylight had other things to think about apart from astonishing patches of green popping up in the desert camp. The plastic surgeon sat out in his garden not in the cool of the evening but in between the long bouts of surgery, when the sun was at its brightest and hottest. The surgical theatres at Bastion were air-conditioned, sometimes a little too efficiently, and they got chilly after hours of operating. Patients had to be warmed up once they came back to the wards. Everyone shivered under their cotton scrubs by the time they had finished, and it was worst of all for the plastic surgeon. Back at home the theatres where he stood for hours and mended burns injury were kept really warm – 28 degrees minimum – all the time, because the cold is bad for burns patients. So he was used to working in the warmth, flourished in it. When he went out into the garden in the glare of the sun, it was to warm himself up properly and to see how his plants were doing, the bright hope of green in a leaf, not the dull khaki of uniform T-shirts or the laundry-bleached blue of theatre scrubs or the base yellow of the limb disposal bags lined up against a wall.[18]

Some things were beyond the power of a garden, though. A MERT team leader walked into the hospital at Bastion to do the paperwork for a job they had done earlier that day. It had been extremely tough – both legs lost, lines inserted wherever there was room, the casualty as far gone as humanly possible – but they had brought him some of the way back, and all the way to the operating theatre, so really a job gone quite well. She moved from the heat of the open ground into the immediate cool of the hospital, the ringing in her ears from the noise and vibration of the helicopter cabin diminishing with each step. As she pushed open the trauma unit door, file tucked under her arm, the silence halted her in her tracks. No noise in the trauma bay, no doctors bent over her patient, calling to each other, giving updates, no clattering instruments, monitors, machines. Instead they were stood back, stopped, and the team leader was quietly explaining that they should put down whatever they were holding, and that care was to cease.[19] The rest was silence. And in the trauma bay next door a team still worked, desperate to ignore the silence that had descended just behind the curtain a few feet from their own efforts to battle back.

Silence. When, no matter what they did, the cascade could not be stopped and the poison was everywhere, when no matter how much blood had been pumped back in it simply flowed back out, when nothing anyone was doing seemed to make any difference. Skin cooling, colour fading, eyes losing light, for the last time. Then the moment, the single moment, when the team leader looked at his watch and asked his team to stop, diagnosing and pronouncing death as quietly as any priest at a committal. Heads shaking, pleading for another two minutes, perhaps something else, something different, but there was never another two minutes, and at the back of the collective mind there was relief that it was over, and that someone else had had the calm and courage to make the call. Eventually knowing that there was nothing more. A moment of reflection, a shift into stillness, for everyone's sake. Silence. Much quieter voices began the paper trail that followed the dead, as dressings were applied to wounds stitched up as a courtesy, lines left in, gloves and aprons ripped off and binned for burning. Many of the staff were emergency specialists from home, so they had seen death before and knew what was expected from them. Waiting until the other bays are empty so the body could be discreetly wheeled away, the blood mopped off the floor, the supply cabinets restocked for next time.

Those waiting outside pacing the corridors – some of them friends, often from the same unit – were told, and sometimes the surgeon could not help but notice as he told them that their desperate faces were red and abraded from the same blast that had blown away their comrade.[20] A *Minimise* protocol was announced. *Minimise* meant a death at the hospital, so no internet, no mobile phone use, total communication blackout to prevent the information getting out before the next of kin had been told. It could last a few hours or days, until everyone was properly accounted for. Across the desert in the American military camps it was called the River City protocol (from the musical *The Music Man*: 'Ya got trouble, right here in River City …'). At Bastion everyone knew when someone had died at the hospital: one word, *Minimise,* and silence fell across the huge camp.

Bastion always had its own mortuary. It was not particularly large and in the early years, before the hard-build, had been a tent with limited lighting, the shadowy canvas folds absorbing all other sounds, cloaking itself around the black plastic body bag on the table at its centre. As Bastion modernised, so did its mortuary, becoming a refrigerated hard-built unit, with its own staff. Access was always tightly controlled as the administration and preparation of death and its consequences were undertaken. Because the deaths of British nationals meant a long journey halfway around the world, across the continents, an international death certificate was required. Certification was done by the most senior doctor, usually the medical director, at the hospital – the one who had been at Musgrave Park and Kosovo, and had deployed to Iraq and had signed a hundred certificates there, and then many more at Bastion.

It was a task he undertook alone. Just him, and the dead, in the tent and then in the hard-build mortuary. Sometimes there was so very little left of the body that all he could write on the death certificate was 'Total body disruption'. He knew that there was nothing about his experience that was worth the learning, so no junior surgeons or doctors came in with him; he never whispered a short lecture about certification in the mortuary but instead covered it in other training sessions, in other places. There was usually something to send home and bury but sometimes not much. When Richard Hillary was burned to death training to fly night fighters in 1944, there was nothing left that distinguished his body from the wreckage of the aircraft, and so, like all the other aircrew whose remains were nothing but ash, the coffin carried into church for his funeral was full of sand. Something was better than nothing. Sand is still used today to make up for the weight of a remnant body in a coffin. Death at Bastion. Dust and fines and sand.

9

History

THE YEAR WHEN THIS BOOK was commissioned, 2014, marked not only the withdrawal of the last British service personnel from Afghanistan but also the centenary of the outbreak of the First World War, in the autumn of 1914. Before we can go forward, we have to go back to understand why all this has happened before. The movement of clinical capability to a point further forward than ever thought humanly possible, the transformation of British military medicine out where the battles are fought, the unexpected survival of significant numbers of human beings, saved, treated, made strong enough to travel all the way home.

And then we need to go back also to understand that all of this failed, how all those journeys racing out to the point of wounding to bring back living casualties with such extraordinary skill were made meaningless after the end of the First World War in 1918. How an extraordinary infrastructure, with magnificent commitment and potential to solve problems and ease lives, was destroyed – not forgotten, or insufficiently funded – but destroyed. How what was left was a broken road, going nowhere, and littered along it were hundreds of thousands of men living broken, silent, pain-wracked, foreshortened lives. This is what I talk to my colleagues in Blast Injury about, and it is alarming how much they recognise as having direct parallels today.

If we go back and look at the amputee cohort from the First World War, we see that it is huge – 41,000 men with one or more limbs missing, enough to fill a medium-size football stadium. A century ago, medics at all levels, surgeons to stretcher-bearers, got better at saving the lives of those brought in from the shell craters of No Man's Land, particularly those with their legs or arms blasted by artillery shell fragments and shrapnel. Death rates for the biggest killer, femoral fracture – the smashing of the big bone in the thigh – came down from 50 per cent to 10 per cent between 1916 and 1918. Practice makes experts, experts save lives: everything that was done at Bastion had been done before in field hospitals along the Western Front.

There were new forms of expertise as well. Orthopaedic surgeons, part of a relatively new specialism, came to the First World War and brought with them a whole new mindset that would transform the prospects of those with limb loss, at least for a while. Orthopaedists, then as now, think about humans as locomotor *systems* – not just bone by bone, limb isolated from limb, but whole systems. Damage one component and it affects everything else, for ever. The roots of modern orthopaedics grew from the treatment of children, or as late Victorian England put it, 'malformed' children. Children with congenital deformation of their spines or skeletal systems, children left twisted and misshapen by polio, rickets and other diseases, or by malnutrition. Children are all little system, too small to pick out any one thing, and the surgeon looking down at their malformation has no choice but to see the interconnectedness of it all. If he makes one small adjustment, it will allow somewhere else to be straightened out, and so on, and all while their patient still has growing to do. But get the small adjustment wrong, see it only in isolation, and then malformation becomes disability and everything gets worse.

In one of those useful things that makes the historian's life so much easier, one man was largely responsible for the creation of modern orthopaedics. Robert Jones studied surgery at the end of the nineteenth century with his uncle in Liverpool, where their practice was full of dockers injured at work. Moving into his own practice, Jones assumed responsibility for the workers digging the Manchester Ship Canal. Both of these sites were heavily industrialised, labour-intensive and dangerous – much like the First World War – and Jones devised systems designed to treat hundreds of patients as quickly and as effectively as possible. At the same time he became involved with the treatment of malformed children, founding first a hospital and then a network of medical facilities for their treatment. But most of all, he brought it all together. Locomotor systems, malformed children, industrial injury, surgery and rehabilitation. An entire system, proven to work in numbers, and with young, inspired staff ready to take on the world.

And this is what Jones sent to the Western Front when he was appointed Director of Military Orthopaedics in March 1916. His young cadre of orthopaedic surgeons worked in the new field hospitals, specially built within earshot of the guns and the line, with emergency departments, pre- and post-operative wards, everything that was needed to ensure that lives were saved and kept saved for the next stage of the journey. And no matter the numbers, no matter that they stood at the operating table for hour after hour, cutting away whatever they couldn't save, for the orthopaedic surgeons it was always about the locomotor system: still about anatomy, not just a foot, or a hand or an arm or a leg, or legs, still about restoration, whatever was required in order to fit men again for work in front-line trenches or a new kind of life at home.[1]

At home there were 20,000 orthopaedic beds by the end of 1916 to cope with the surge of casualties returning with upper and lower limb damage, and a flagship unit, at Shepherd's Bush, specially built, a system in itself, with operating theatres, gymnasiums, workshops and soldiers working there to build and repair their own prosthetics, and build and repair those of their comrades. So much of what we have now came from then:

inside the limb-makers' workshops [...] the patient was made to try the limb in the rough by walking at first between two parallel wooded rails on which he could rest his hands. At each of these rails was a large looking-glass in which he could see how he walked, so that he might correct errors.[2]

All over the country other specialist units were part of the system, needed by a cohort of patients that make today's surgeons shudder.[3] In one article written for *The Lancet* a surgeon called for improvements in stump surgery 'based on the experience of 2,000 consecutive cases' that he had seen in a fifteen-month period.[4] Every surgeon working on limb casualty was aware that this was only a beginning, that what they were seeing would become the great aftermath of disability and pain.[5]

All the young surgeons who had watched over dimly lit field hospital wards, who had written hurried articles back to journals so that others might learn as they had, came back to Britain determined that their new knowledge should not go to waste. They tended their military patients and spread the word about the value of what had been learned, but also about how much more still needed doing. On 10 April 1919 one young orthopaedic surgeon came to the Imperial College of Science. He stood and spoke to an audience of civilian medics and engineers in a lecture theatre that is still in use today, where I have given lectures. He used a lantern show (an early version of PowerPoint) to show photographs of the improvements in the care of his military patients with lower limb fractures, and a cinematograph (video embedded in PowerPoint) to show his patients six months after they left the hospital.

Down the corridor, on the same afternoon, Imperial staff and students could also go and hear one of the young surgeons from the facial repair unit at Sidcup. Led by the plastic surgeon Harold Gillies, Sidcup was Britain's first hospital specialising in the repair of both the hard and soft tissues of the face. Like

Jones, Gillies had brought together specialists from the world of plastic surgery and dental surgery in an entirely new system dedicated to meeting the challenge of facial wounds. In what was probably a much more gruesome presentation for the lay viewer, surgeons from Sidcup presented their lantern show of cases of

> patients who had mutilating wounds of the face, especially loss of the nose or great part of the jaw [...] the contrast between the results obtained by the ingenious grafting of bone, cartilage and soft parts, and the previous conditions seen in the photographs or casts was particularly striking.[6]

It wasn't a coincidence that these speakers came to South Ken. The First World War was the making of Imperial.[7] It was less than ten years old, and made up of a variety of institutes operating together rather too loosely. It might not have survived the exodus of staff and students to serve in the military (a third of the staff and half the students) had the remainder not proved their versatility and utility to the government during the war itself. So when the survivors came back, they found an institution that had consolidated itself around multidisciplinary projects and a shared experience of finding themselves necessary to their country, either at the front or in the laboratory.[8]

The First World War should have been the making of orthopaedics, and plastics as well. The two newest surgical specialisms were poised to meet the continuing challenge of soldiers in the process of restoration, and to apply their new expertise in the civilian sector. But by 1925 everything that they had meant during the war and that day in a lecture theatre in South Kensington had gone. Understanding why is fundamental, because only then can we understand how it might happen again, and only then can we understand just how much was lost.[9]

The most powerful institution in British medicine in the

early twentieth century was the Royal College of Surgeons. It was dominated by general surgeons – who did surgery on whatever was required of them, hard or soft tissue – and the generalist view did not equate to the orthopaedists' view. There were no systems in the general surgeon's world, only limbs and organs. It was not the job of the surgeon to become involved with systems, or with aftercare and its providers. Surgery was always at the heart of medical care by general surgeons. Surgeons who operated differently diluted the status of their practice, challenged its supremacy. That affected everything, including their fee structure. New consultancies could not be allowed to rise, and so they were not.

The support of the Royal College of Surgeons, irrelevant in wartime because of the emergency, was essential in the period afterwards, and it was withdrawn. Without it, plans for education and research into the aftermath of locomotor injury could not be realised. Wards closed, units closed, all of them: the research laboratory–workshop at Roehampton in 1924, even Shepherd's Bush by 1925. Patients were moved to units within large general hospitals, with excellent medical provision but no prospect of developing the skills necessary to combat the complex aftermath of pain and dysfunction. The same thing happened with plastic surgery. Harold Gillies, chief surgeon at Sidcup and today internationally recognised as one of the pioneers of modern reconstructive surgery, was demoted back to general surgeon and reduced to 'begging for scraps' of soft tissue repair, mostly closure of wounds, at the end of procedures to keep his plastics skills current.[10]

With the diminution of orthopaedics went everything else: all the physiotherapists, the really expert non-surgeons in the repair of the locomotor system, and also the potential to fix the long-term problems, the ones that they were only just beginning to recognise. The Ministry of Pensions took over much of the management of rehabilitation, and the Haig Fund (later to become the British Legion) filled the gaps in welfare. What had been solid was fractured, dispersed. Patients could find their own way to see surgeons, who might have a small network of therapists they could call on, but mostly they could not. The aftermath became a wilderness, where men stumbled and retreated and where no roads forward could be seen. And this happened not because of money, not through lack of funding, but because of institutions resisting change. People, not money. That's what my colleagues recognise today when I tell them about yesterday, and that's what's worrying.

*

And in the meantime, back to Bastion.

10

Critical Care

The multiply injured soldier has multiple contaminated
wounds, is systemically unwell, immuno-compromised
following massive blood transfusion and requires multi-
system support in a Critical Care environment.[1]

MULTI-SYSTEM SUPPORT. Nursing, in other words. We know
the name and the life story of Harold Gillies, pioneering plastic
surgeon in Britain during the First World War, but we know
almost nothing about the nurses who kept his soldier patients
clean and uninfected and alive, who fed and watered them sip
by sip through shredded mouths and noses, who watched over
them in their pain – who made them strong enough for long
anaesthetics and complex operations. We call this critical care
nursing now and there was a Critical Care ward at Bastion,
next to the pathology lab (good reason for that, see below).

Most of the patients who needed nursing at Bastion were
locals, who went from short stays in Critical Care to the
ordinary wards until they could be moved on. Nurses, like
everyone else, relied on Terps for their daily communication
with these patients, but usually, once the emergencies were
passed, this was (mostly) straightforward. In some ways it
could be easier than nursing at home. When I asked a senior
nurse what she particularly remembered about this kind of
work, she said Antibiotics. Her Afghan patients responded to

antibiotics much more quickly than her patients back in the UK. No matter how serious their infections (and Afghanistan had myriad ways to infect the human body), a short course of antibiotics and they were usually all cleared up in forty-eight hours. No multiple courses and no allergies. So much easier than nursing in an antibiotic-resistant population. Just an observation, no control trial to test her hypothesis but something unexpected to appreciate.

So it wasn't the long-stay patients who posed the greatest challenges to Bastion's nursing staff; it was the short-stay ones. British military casualties who came in on MERT, who were revived in the trauma bays and had damage control surgery in the operating theatre only stayed in Critical Care until they could be moved back to the UK, usually twenty-four hours or less. Definitive surgery, the kind that needed microscopes and more kit than even Bastion could provide, could only be done at home, so in the meantime, critical care.

The meantime at Bastion was something more than holding the patient steady until the transport came for them. The meantime was when those watching most closely came to understand the exact terms of the deal for life that had just been done in MERT and the trauma bay and the operating theatre. Understanding really meant management of the consequences of the negotiation. The inflammatory storm – the tsunami in the body – receded, leaving behind its wreckage and poison throughout the body of the patient. Nurses worked in its wake, clearing a space so that later others could go on working. Starting with those multiple contaminated wounds.

Much of the nurses' time, unsurprisingly, was taken up with wound care. By the end of 2009 most blast wounds were coming in avulsive, with the soft flesh and all its workings blasted high up the limb, away from the bone fracture. The surgeons did their best, and when they finished, the wound was swamped with hydrogen peroxide, a last sample was taken for lab tests and then what's left came back to the ward at Bastion for management. Avulsive wounds bleed, and when they've been stopped from bleeding, they exude another liquid – exudate, as if they are sweating heavily under extreme stress ('exudate' comes from the Latin word *exudare*, meaning 'to sweat'). Nurses see it in wards back home all the time from ordinary wounds and surgical repairs, just not as much of it. There was so much on the ward at Bastion.

Exudate can be clear, or opaque, amber or grey-green, odourless or foul. There needs to be just the right amount of it to indicate healing.[2] Exudate keeps wounds moist and gently swills good stuff like proteins and growth factors and nutrients around a wound site, which encourages it to get on with healing. A good wound looks glossy, with small amounts of exudate visible and neat edges left behind by the surgeon. Too little exudate (scaly skin, dressing sticking to the wound) means that the body can no longer produce it and that something much more serious is going wrong, systemically, such as shock or severe dehydration. Too much, and the problem is local, at the wound face itself: disordered inflammatory mechanisms make the actual wound eat into previously undamaged tissue, and there's little enough of that to spare on an avulsive wound. Too much was usually the problem at Bastion.

Too much exudate, like sweat stains on a shirt, soaks through ordinary dressings. When exudate gets to the outside layer (with the uncharacteristically dramatic medical name of strikethrough), then any antimicrobial properties of the dressing, the barrier between air germs and vulnerable wound sites, is lost. It's the same principle for when the blood or gunk from a scrape on your knee soaks through your plaster: it means the plaster (dressing) is useless. It should be taken off, till the bleeding or seeping has stopped, and then a new one put on. But in military wounds, especially avulsive blast wounds, the exudate keeps coming, and if it isn't kept clean, it starts to smell like the nastiest sweat imaginable, and you can't keep taking off the plasters and putting on new ones because it means more chance of infection, less chance of healing, and it hurts. It really hurts.

So there's a twenty-first-century solution: negative pressure wound therapy. It sounds like a physics solution, and it is. Dressings are applied over the wound site, packing down right to the wound bed. The dressings are gauzy material, and impregnated with antimicrobials. If it's a deep wound, thick pads of the gauze are used, pushed down inch by inch – not too tight, not compacted, just enough to fill, with the tail end left outside the wound, so nurses never forget there are rolls deep in there, and eventually all of them will be taken out. But it's wonderful stuff, so if they get it right they can leave it in for as long as necessary (sometimes two weeks even). The gauze is absorbent, permeable, but very gently so, like lung tissue, so you'd hardly notice as the liquid passes through it safely. And then a drain tube, with a round transparent pad at one end, is settled on the dressing, with all the edges sealed around the wound. At the other end of the tube is a fat plastic box that contains the compression pump. Turn it on, and the negative pressure created by the gentle force of the dressing absorption meets the positive pressure from the pump and the exudate is drawn away up the tube, into a collection canister, almost silently – just a slight, constant hum from the compression unit, one of those excellent sounds medics like to notice on a trauma ward. And for the patient, no ripped dressings, no more smell, no more lying in bed knowing almost nothing for certain except that the smell of rot comes from themselves.

Turn on the pumps, let them manage the wound and then step back to see more of the consequences of the deal. Beyond the wounds, a systemically unwell patient. Life now, but of very poor quality in the meantime. A hungry, degraded body that had started to lose muscle mass almost the moment it was injured, because it had almost no other reserves. Soldiers were usually super-fit, with almost no body fat, as a result of exercising compulsively and competitively as a way to pass the time. Many of them had been out in forward positions for months living off rations, with not much fresh fruit – plenty of tinned, but not a great diet considering the physical demands and the stress. And even though now they are stable, lying in one spot, not moving and mostly asleep, they use up energy just by being, by staying alive, by surviving on the spot, no movement forward. So nourishment is as necessary as the oxygen in the ventilator, the negative pressure pump on the dressing and the antibiotics in the intravenous lines.[3]

Not just hungry. Something much worse than just hungry. The body in the bed might be still and sleeping, but inside it has begun to turn on itself, feeding off whatever it can find, because it needs the energy to make it to the next pulse beat. And although the inflammatory storm has passed, inflammatory responses are still there, now chronic and dangerous. There are no more dead cells to eat, so now they start on live ones because they can't tell the difference any more. Exudate is full of protein, and if the little collection vessel attached to the tube is filling up and emptying regularly, it's good in one way but it means that the patient is loosing fluid and protein.

Here are the technical terms for what happens when a traumatised body starts to feed on itself. They all begin with 'hyper' – and that's never a good thing. *Hypermetabolic*: galloping energy consumption where muscle tissue is broken down directly and feeds into the bloodstream for energy for the cells. *Hyperglycaemia:* traumatic diabetes, where insulin levels are out of control every which way, damaging liver and kidneys. *Hyperlactatemia:* acid levels soaring because there is less oxygen because of bleeding, more energy needed from everywhere else, stress hormones, flooding in because this is extreme trauma, and poison from infections. Here's a non-technical term to describe what is happening: a cannibal chemical soup that is gradually eating the human from within to survive and killing them at the same time.

So in Critical Care new intravenous lines, preferably directly into the stomach or, if there were complications, straight into one of the large veins in the chest or the arm. And before inserting the new line, nurses make complicated calculations and measurements (or 'defined algorithms, tables and equations') – how much of muscles that lifted rifles or dug out mines has now wasted away – to work out what exactly needs to be put back in. Essentially proteins, glucose, fats, amino acids, immune supplements, even fibre, to prevent constipation, which everyone can do without. The jury's still out on fish oils, but fatty acids might be a way to help and they don't seem to do any harm. And perhaps, when the lines are in and the calculations are done, nurses can watch and see some improvement, life a little better.

The easiest and most immediate way for nurses to make their patients' lives better was to treat their pain. They had general anaesthesia to start with, on the way into surgery. Then, if they were awake, normally or post-operatively, questions about pain (pain treatment always starts with questions) and then drugs and plenty of them: synthetic opioids (opiates only if the compound derives actually from the natural source of opium, the poppy, grown all over the world throughout human history, quite a bit of it in Afghanistan, oh the irony). Opioids work best on acute pain, particularly post-surgical pain. Lots of that at Bastion. So opioids are the best response overall. They bind to specific receptors in the nervous system and quieten them down. The pain itself is reduced, and the sensations of pain in body and mind are also lessened. The downside of opioids it that they knock the patient out, or make them very woozy. And they aren't site-specific. Opioids are a whole-body response, when something that targets more carefully would really help too.

Site-specific pain relief is called regional (as opposed to general) anaesthesia. Regional implies a bigger area to be treated than local anaesthesia, which is for smaller things such as single teeth. The anaesthetist who kept the patient under for their surgery comes back to the ward. They have ultrasound machines which help them locate the exact nerve that needs blocking, and once they've done that, they insert a needle, with a small plastic catheter (about the size of angel hair spaghetti) threaded through it. Needle in, needle out, catheter inserted.

Dressing on, please, nurse. And then the catheter is connected to a pump full of medication and slowly starts to dispense it directly where it is needed. It blocks the nerve sending the screaming signals from the injury to the brain. Simple. Put the drugs where the pain is, where it starts, stop it going all the way to the point where the chemical soup is started – the hormones, the stress, the fear. There are lots of advantages to nerve blocks, and fewer side-effects. Opioids cause drowsiness, and they usually cause constipation, itchiness and they can make the patient feel sick. The lack of drowsiness means the patient can move more, maybe even have a little physiotherapy to get their systems going.

And just like negative pressure wound dressings, medics can use as many nerve blocks as necessary to prevent pain. Multiple injuries, multiple nerve blocks, multiple ways and means. Nerve blocks, lined up somewhere clean and convenient, not anywhere where the bones are fractured, so they can be managed without causing more pain and damage. And not too high on the body, or too low: in fact, just right. An amputation of the leg or legs, they get an epidural (catheter in the spine, a nerve block too, one of the first to be used frequently). Abdominal or pelvic injury, along with upper limb injury, and they get a nerve block catheter just above the collarbone. Sometimes it was the shredding of blast injury that made nerve block use too difficult, so then it was back to general analgesia, usually via patient-controlled analgesia (PCA) pumps – patient feels pain, patient depresses button on pump, patient gets more painkiller. The first jokes soldiers made after they found themselves in Critical Care were usually about the PCA pumps – threatening to take more if their mates came in and bored them or cried, miming multiple pumps of the drugs and lolling dramatically.

So more pumps and machines round the bed and catheters to monitor for the nerve blocks for the patients who stayed awake. All those instructions in journal articles about keeping the catheter site clean – those are for nurses, who have to go in and look closely at every entry point for signs of redness, swelling, with the patient inhaling sharply when nurses gently touch it with their very gloved hands. Unmonitored, infection can bite deep and quick; in epidurals a dirty catheter is a fast lane to neurological infections such as meningitis. Epidural catheters warrant their own chart, filled out hourly, with things like drug levels in the block, and a pain score; if there's a severe, unexpected infection, this is where it will be seen. If the pain starts to come back, then get the anaesthetist to come and up the dose. And nurses know their way around the pumps the patients use themselves, how to turn them on and off and up or down, and how to change the batteries. It's a lot to remember, but remember how much easier it is now the patients aren't battered into submission by strong IV medications, usually opioids, and anything that helps keep them off ventilators is most welcome. And there's science to back all of this up.[4] Wherever the nurse is, whatever they are watching, if in doubt, labs – skin, blood, catheter tips, anything, test it all, again, even if they've tested the regulation amount of times already. That's why the pathology lab, where the testing could be done, was so close by at Bastion.

Even though nerve blocks and epidurals have been common for years in civilian hospitals, the tented military hospital just couldn't provide a sufficiently sterile environment for their use. But the hard-build made of hermetically sealed Portakabin units could. Throw in portable ultrasound machines and really good catheters, and experience in their use, and nerve blocks came to Bastion in time for 2009, when they would be really needed. Here's that underlying principle of military medicine again – move clinical capability as far forward as it will go, even if sometimes it means waiting for a hard-build. Because it means that next time they will have worked out how to use nerve blocks in a more austere environment, as well as even smaller ultrasound, different bacteria-resistant catheter tips, cold storage to keep them all in, all ready to go. Clinical capability forward: bring the hospital to the patient, in a hard-build or a helicopter, bring as much of the hospital at home to the patient in the war zone. Do it quickly, do it well and (hopefully) everything is easier the other end.

Military nurses moved quietly around their ward at Bastion, men and women dressed the same in combats but most of the women with the neat bun of hair tucked at the back of their head. It looks like a world away from any other world or any other time, but especially from that of their predecessors in the First World War, who wore the uncomfortable starched dresses and white veils and remonstrations from Sister if the laundry hadn't been done well or frequently enough. But whatever the uniform, nursing military trauma across a century is in essence the same: watching the wound, watching the wounded, feeling strongly about those whom they will never actually meet in person.[5] Hearing without listening the change in breath sounds, seeing mates gathered at the doorway, knowing when to call a surgeon, when to change the negative pressure pump. Better scent receptors than the finest perfumer, and knowing how to keep a smile even for those who might not yet be able to see it. Seeing problems no one else can see, and finding solutions. Not solutions that involve algorithms, tables and equations – so no research trial or journal article, or points on the promotion scale – but still solutions that make things easier, better, not just for their patient but also for the patient's kin, who wait along the road for their loved one to be strong enough to reach them.

Patient diaries are just such a solution to a range of problems for nurses across Critical Care, whether civilian or military. And they are the answer to a hard question, the one about what happened while their patient was asleep. In 2008 a nurse arrived at Bastion. The long wait in the aircraft hangar, then the tactical landing in Afghanistan, bumping down on the runway in total darkness, the dust and fines, then the drive to the hospital. But the hospital was like nothing that he had experienced on his tours in Iraq. The ITU (Critical Care) looked like it did at home: the same artificial light, the same air-conditioning, a world within a world, quiet, safety. A ward round, wounds and the wounded explained to the staff caring for them (patients rarely sufficiently awake) and then swiftly patients gone, flying back home, someone new, sedated and ventilated, in their bed. Most unconscious until Birmingham, and he knew this was going to be a problem. He'd watched patients wake on an ITU ward, saw their panic at where they were, not knowing why they were as they were, and the deep stress inflicted on them by the process. ITU staff tried to explain, but shifts and bleeps got in the way. As ITUs became more advanced, so did a condition known as ITU-PTSD – the stress induced, post-traumatically, by not knowing what has happened to the patient during the hours and days that are missing from their memory.

How much worse, he thought, would this be for the soldier who fell in the desert, was swooped away by MERT, saved and nursed at Bastion, flown half a continent away and then woken, not with their unit around them dusty and shouting, but their family, strained and weeping. At home ITU-PTSD was being mitigated by something very simple: a diary. In it nurses wrote down the things they would say if their unconscious patient could hear them.[6] Not a medical record – that was something separate – a diary. Of pain, of sleep, of dreams, of weather outside the window, of visitors, of watching, of time passing. They should have patient diaries at Bastion, where the moments in between the explosions and echoes could be recorded, sorted and retold.

The nurse had been working in a health service in one form or another for long enough to know that this sort of thing was better done himself, improvised rather than waiting for clearance. So when he went home on leave he designed a notebook that could be a diary, and took it to a printer, and paid £180 to have several hundred copies made. Very simple, A5 size. On the cardboard cover were basic details such as name and date of admittance, and inside three columns: Date & Time, Narrative and Signature. And then, when the boxes of diaries arrived back from the printer, he went round all his colleagues and handed them out and explained how they worked.

Some of them already knew because they'd seen them in Critical Care at home, but everyone said *what a brilliant idea,* right from the outset. A civilian innovation adapted and improved in their little ward in a hospital in the desert. Watching their wounded became something different, something better. They pulled up a chair and dug out a pen (often from where some of them had stuck it in the bun at the back of their head) and remembered what they'd just done, how they might have told the patient quietly about it even though he was unconscious, but now they could tell him in a way that he might eventually know and understand. How much blood he'd been given, that they had donated their own blood to the hospital's supply and now it flowed through his veins. That, even though they were supposed to have gone off duty, they had stayed on at his side. That someone had been watching him, never a moment alone, until they handed him over to the next watcher, and they to the next, until he was awake.

The patient diary system started small but soon spread, and the medical officer in charge recognised how well they worked, so they became part of the official system, part of the standard paperwork, part of a training course even. That sort of thing usually took years and committees and meetings – in Bastion, double-quick smart, something that works, use it. They were one of those things that, as soon as they were told about them, everyone just knew were a good thing. Word spread out of the hospital and up the runway to where the MERT crew lived. Just like everyone who handed over a patient they had kept alive, MERT crew wanted to know what happened to the soldier rushed into a trauma bay. So nurses on the ward let them in to see their patients, to read the diaries and to understand what had happened afterwards, and then they asked if they too could make entries, so the soldier would know he had not just been slung in and out, but that many people had looked after him in flight, that he had been fought for, every second, every pulse beat, all the resources and effort they had to offer.[7] And somehow filling out the diaries helped the MERT crew too, although one RAF nurse remembered always walking away quickly from the ward, tears on her face, which she wiped away as she found her way back to her quarters to make ready to go out again.

Friends too. Diaries gave them something to do when they came to see their friend, who couldn't hear them or reply, so they didn't just have to stand there and worry whether they were allowed to touch him nervously on his shoulder or if they would mess up the lines running in and out of him, or bother a nurse to ask. They could just pick up the diary and find a pen and sit down and write, including the time and the date. This could sometimes go wrong. The plastic surgeon was on the ward checking on a patient and watched as a group of soldiers sat by their unconscious, heavily sedated, battered comrade and started to write in the diary. After a while they realised it wasn't who they thought it was, so one of them quickly wrote 'Sorry mate, we thought it was someone else. Get well soon anyway.' (This was told as a joke by the Bastion medics but is testimony to something more sobering. Soldiers could be living at a patrol base cheek by jowl with each other for months, sharing immediately every detail of each other's lives, but blast injury could render them unrecognisable one to the other, swollen, battered, anonymous, a remnant.) Diaries went home in the paperwork folder on the Critical Care Air Support Team flights between Afghanistan and Birmingham, where nurses and flight crew added their thoughts and messages. Entry by entry the diaries grew as a record, beyond the medical, of the human beneath the lines.

Pen to paper, important for everyone, making a record. When patients made it out of the trauma bays and the operating theatre, patients who by rights shouldn't have, nurses took a red marker pen and drew a small red heart next to their names on the admissions board. These were the first visible notations given to unexpected survivors by anyone at Bastion – the journal articles describing the condition in technical medical detail hadn't really got going – and they made for a good, easily read answer to the hard question of what happened to the patient next.

*

On 2 January 2011 nurses in the Critical Care ward at Bastion began a patient diary for Scott Meenagh. Scott had no memory of what had happened to him after the first forty seconds of the MERT flight in the Chinook, so the diary pages (four of them, double-sided, even though he was at Bastion for less than twenty-four hours) told him what had happened there, words from medics, MERT crew and his comrades who had held it together and got him on board the helicopter.

One of the paramedics visited him in Critical Care:

> Scott, Get well Soon! I came to get you and load you on the RAF MERT Chinook. You are in great hands now and will be in the future as you get back in it!

One of the nurses who had attended him and the other casualties from his unit in the trauma bay came through to the ward:

> I was in ED [Emergency Department] this morning co-ordinating the help you and your colleagues needed. This was a real privilege to do. You may have dark days ahead but I am sure your friends and family will get you through the months to come.

After them came his nurses, pulling up a chair next to his bed, finding a pen, starting to write to the patient whom they would never actually meet:

> Hi Scott; I looked after you when you first came to the Critical Care unit from the operating theatre. We kept you asleep and gave you lots of pain killers. Keeping you asleep was difficult at first because you are such a big bloke. Anyway, all the best and stay strong.

The hospital padre, who had waited in the ward all day, as he did whenever casualties were admitted, wrote:

> Scott, from the time of this incident itself you've received all the care it was possible to give. As people have visited you today, I've prayed for you and those involved. My prayers for your recovery and return to full health as you face the future.

No matter that he couldn't hear them, a steady stream of visitors had sat down at his bedside to write in the diary, from his CO ('The thoughts and prayers of all at 2 Para are with you') to his mates. 'That's airborne' was one response to the news of how he had applied his own tourniquets. And from a particularly close friend in his unit who badly wanted him to know that he had been there, as long as he could, although he too was on his way home:

> Scotty, it's [...]. How's it going brother. Am just going on R&R and I'll come to Brummy [Birmingham] to visit you. We're [...] still going on that holiday we always planned on a beach somewhere.
> Am gonna sit here now till they kick me out and mumble crap in your ear. I'll probably bore you but your just going to have to listen. See you in Birmingham Meenagee, love your brother [...].

And from a MERT crewman, the first real statement that Scott's life would now be something very different from what it had been that morning:

> We brought you back from Bastion and now the best we have is for you. Good luck for your onward journey and beyond.

11

Critical Care Air Support Team (CCAST)

So here we are [...] halfway home, somewhere in the sky.

Patient diary entry, 14 February 2011, 0130 Zulu time

GOING HOME. British casualties were moved as soon as the staff in Critical Care had made and held them strong enough for the journey. What they had at Bastion was damage limitation. What they needed from now on was definitive repair, and that could only be done at home. And besides, the next patient was bumping down at Nightingale, needing the bed and the medics waiting in the trauma bay.[1] So those who could be moved were. Surgeries finished, transfusions holding, breathing steady, wounds packed tight, pain and infections managed. A different kind of movement of clinical capability – expertly managed transitions, skills designed not to waste any of the work that has gone before. For the time being.

The time being was a journey across a continent, three thousand miles, from Afghanistan to Britain.[2] Along the time being, the patient was carried in huge aircraft, high above the planet, the C-17 Globemasters. Another world from Bastion, another life – going to another life. A critical care support team sustaining them in the air, like MERT, only much less bumpy. A medical team of six: one nurse per patient (and on CCAST the team leader was always one of these nurses), and one spare who went where they were needed, a Critical Care anaesthetic consultant, a trainee, an RAF medic and a medical technology specialist. Aircrew: a loadmaster who saw to what was carried whether it breathed or not, maintenance crew and three pilots, two flying, one spare resting, at the front. Sustaining life one pulse beat at a time as the miles flew past below. Surround and sustain.

When the 9-Liner was received at Bastion, the message about the wounding went out along the entire chain of care, from MERT quarters, through the resus bays in the hospital at Bastion, the hospital at Birmingham and the headquarters of the CCAST at Brize Norton – beepers going off thousands of miles apart within fifteen minutes of the blast of the IED. The aim for every critically ill patient was to get them home within forty-eight hours, but it was often much less than that. Severely injured patients could be ten hours in surgery and then less than a day on the ward. Scott Meenagh's patient dairy covered only one day in what had become the first of the rest of his life: explosions, surgery, on to Critical Care at 1400 hrs on 25 January 2011, then off it by midnight to fly home.[3]

Even at maximum capacity during the hammering of the hospital in 2010 – five separate beds bearing five separate critically ill patients, five separate teams, one for each plus a stretcher case and walking wounded – this system (the air-bridge, they called it) worked properly throughout. It was once reorganised in 2010, because of the ash cloud from Iceland's Eyjafjallajökull which seeded the sky with volcanic dust and fines and grounded all the planes over Europe, no matter who they carried.[4] A CCAST flight was the last flight to land in the UK before the grounding, getting special permission to do so. And because no one knew how long the ban would last, a back-up was implemented that put a CCAST crew and aircraft in southern Spain because flights were possible across southern Europe. But it never came to that. Along the air-bridge, people were where they said they would be, when they were supposed to be, and they knew what to expect when they got there.

*

When CCAST landed at Bastion, they didn't wait for their patient to be brought to them. From the moment the patient was prepared to leave his bed in Critical Care, he belonged to CCAST. Patient and machines. The patient they collected from the ward at Bastion was all lines, pumps, tubes, plastic bags, and none could be disconnected. CCAST arrived in the ward, and the consultant and the team leader nurse moved to the patient. They carried a heavy ventilator and monitors on thick black shoulder straps, and usually they had their own negative pressure wound therapy pumps (always in short supply at Bastion, and they didn't want to let them go). A trolley with a stretcher slid into its side rails was lined up alongside the patient. On the stretcher was a vacuum mattress, like a flat square beanbag, where the air could be pumped in or out, moulding around the patient, especially helpful in the case of spinal injury, fractures and newly amputated limbs. Over that was an absorbent sheet for drawing up blood and fluids. At the top was a head-up backrest that kept the head raised at a 30-degree angle, helping to promote lung function, even if the patient was ventilated.

'Transferring' was called. All the lines and pumps were switched from the ward machines to their CCAST travel equivalent: 'flick and click' they used to call it, right first time on all of them. Then the patient was lifted over on to the stretcher. Another absorbent blanket was put on top of them and then a specially designed harness was strapped over everything, holding each limb in place like a black starfish, so nothing moved when it wasn't supposed to. It was hard to see the human at all now, just quarters of body skin held together by nylon webbing and lines. A spoken handover, along with the paperwork that accompanied the patient all the way home: X-ray films, bloodwork, medical records (usually on a CD), the patient's diary, the patient's passport (theoretically there were immigration checks on arrival, although they never actually took place).

Then as one, they moved. One nurse did nothing but check each line as they transferred, and it needed to be a nurse who didn't mind shouting Stop!, being impolite about tangles, keeping things on track. Then into the back of a military ambulance, line by line, the stretcher slid out of the trolley rails on to a rack in the vehicle. A mile or so, at 15 m.p.h. – no faster, no matter what – to the runway where the transporter plane waits, then unloading, line by line, with eyes never leaving the points where machine meets human. Then slide out the stretcher again, up the ramp, on to the plane, sliding it into a bed frame clipped in on board, arranging the machines around it, line by line, no snagging on the stanchions and framework inside the aircraft. Stop. Check the lines, eyes on the patient, ready to go.

If the CCAST team ever had time to look up as they approached the aircraft, they would have seen a huge machine – the C-17 is not called the Globemaster for nothing – filling their vision waiting to take off. The first war artist who went to Bastion called the giant air transporter 'resplendent', like a cathedral, a huge vaulted space, lit to its roof, even though the inside looked like it was made of Meccano. The floor space is massive and square, wheels in blisters bulging along the rear sides out of the way. It isn't just used to carry the casualties – one time the CCAST crew watched as a bulldozer bumbled its way out and down the ramp and set off along the runway to whoever had ordered it. Then straight away they went up and clipped in their cargo, in the same place, on the same modular system, forgetting what had been there moments before, ready for take-off. An entire Chinook can fit inside, if the rotors are folded up, or a single coffin, covered in a flag, clipped in safely all the way home.

The Globemaster doesn't need a very long runway for take-off – up and off in less than 4,000 feet, ideal for the austere airfield. It goes when it's told. Bastion runway was busy every minute of every hour of every day: transport aircraft, helicopters clattering up and down, and unmarked aircraft and unmanned air vehicles quietly going about their business. The air traffic controllers were the best in the world – no one passed their course unless they scored 80 per cent or higher. The Globemaster did whatever it could to help by making the most of the limited space it occupied.[5] It turned on whatever the aircraft equivalent of a sixpence is, and it could reverse park. It flew stoically for 2,400 nautical miles at 40,000 feet, mountain ranges no problem, with two pilots, one in reserve and a loadmaster. Globemasters were never temperamental, so not much else was needed from ground crew when at rest.

Once the aircraft had cleared the ground and levelled out, beyond the range of enemy attacks, the seatbelt sign went off, the end of tactical darkness, and the lights went up. If there was no turbulence, they could unclip the starfish straps on the trolley, for easier access to the patient. Body armour and helmets off, and the sound of the world high in the sky suddenly bursting over them. Globemaster interiors were noisy, constant, unceasing rattle, clatter, droning hum. Too noisy to speak effectively for hours at a time, so they had their own comms system, headphones and mikes, separate from that of the pilots. This is what they used if they had to confer over their patient, so they left them on all the time and protected their hearing. CCAST crew don't have the tinnitus legacy that many MERT crew have.

Some of the things that might have seemed complicated on board the Globemaster are not. The complex of lines and tubes and pumps swarming over the patient was not affected by the pressure changes of high-altitude flight. Bastion was 3,000 feet above sea level anyway, so patients have been treated at altitude before they ever took off. The cabin was pressurised to 5,000 feet and the difference didn't matter enormously. It didn't mean the medics could ignore the tubes and pumps and lines – they had to keep them clean and wiped, and level and stable, and the flesh around them moist – but they didn't have to worry about the complicated equations about changing oxygen levels at altitude that are in the textbooks. But there are plenty of other things that were complicated enough.

They could move around the patient as necessary. There was plenty of room on the Globemaster, enough for a 360-degree approach, just like MERT, and plenty of light. They needed to take the straps off because their patient needed to be rolled every couple of hours. The vacuum mattress was excellent, but it didn't stop pressure sores, which probably already started back at Bastion from the operating theatre and the ward. One nurse made particular efforts to remember extra gel pads, which she placed around her patients' heads because otherwise they deplaned with blisters or sores and bald spots (occipital alopecia) – extra injuries that no one thanked you for once they got home. There were drugs to be monitored, and adjusted, keeping them down and steady, and dressings to be re-dressed.

Most patients were sedated, so their anaesthetic kept the pain away, but if they stirred or shifted under the blanket, the consultant checked the dosages and adjusted to take them back to comfortable stillness. The few that were awake (and asleep was much easier for the CCAST) got their pain management via epidurals or nerve block catheters or PCAs, which they might be administering themselves with a pump. Only certain models of pump were licensed for use on board military aircraft, in case they interfered with other systems or the other systems on board interfered with them. If there were no nerve blocks, CCAST staff could give analgesia themselves, but they preferred it if the patient came on board with what they needed. And they may very well have needed it. Waking pain could be affected by so many things in flight: the vibration of the aircraft, G-force, air sickness (which could be treated) and plain old-fashioned fear of the moments that were passing and the life to come (which could not).[6] If the flight was long, the analgesia might have started to wear off as it neared the end, so extra medication could be given to help the patient with the manoeuvres of landing, deplaning and transfer. As along the entire length of the pain management pathway, and the CCAST was part of this, medics anticipated pain and its increase or change, and medicated accordingly to stop it happening in the first place, because under-treatment is damaging in the longer term, no matter who or where they are.

But some things were simply too complicated for CCAST. Feeding, for instance. The intravenous feeding tubes inserted in Bastion were removed for the duration of the flight. On CCAST the vibration of the aircraft and any sudden turbulence could cause the fine particles of the food to leak and then, rather than going into the stomach, they went where they shouldn't, such as into the lung tissue, and got infected – micro-aspiration, to give it its proper name. Micro-aspiration causes ventilator-associated pneumonia, and ventilator-associated pneumonia causes death.[7]

On a CCAST flight, even the things they could rely on they were trained not to rely on. Stethoscopes weren't a lot of use – difficult to use with ear protectors, so much background noise and so little human flesh to put them down flat on, since all the useful parts with something to listen to were covered in tape and tubes. The aircraft's background clatter meant it was difficult to hear the bip of the alarm if a ventilator failed, so a light was added that flashed brightly and insistently. Temperature needed to be steady. Fluctuating body temperature indicated changing levels of metabolic disorder, that a body that had just managed to remember how to clot for itself had suddenly forgotten, and that a ravaged immune system was collapsing all over again. So they checked the monitor, constantly. The Globemaster had enough power for all the medical machines on board, and oxygen supplies, but the ventilators ran on batteries anyway, and the staff member responsible checked continually that they were not depleted, and that the store of spare batteries was as per regulations. In theory, the machines could be prone to electrical or magnetic emissions from the aircraft's own power sources. They were tested for airworthiness, but CCAST monitored them, as well as everything else (that's why the technician was there), all the way home.

CCAST had plenty of practice, so, as the rhythm set in amid the clatter of the flight, high above the planet, there was time to reach for the folder with the patient's paperwork in it. The patient diary was there, with the entries from the nurses, and the surgeons and the MERT crew and the friends, so the CCAST added their piece.[8] *You were quiet and steady*, or *You've had a bit of a wobble*, or *We had to give you a little more anaesthetic because the strain had started to show on your face, shadows in the light cutting deeper in the frown.* Not just the medics. One of the nurses went forward and squeezed into the pilots' space with the diary and a pen, and the pilots made their entries. They pasted in a small map and marked out the route they were taking as the continent unfurled beneath their wings: landmass, rivers, mountain ranges, seas. *That's Armenia below us now* (or *Romania* or *Germany* or *Belgium*) and *We came this way because there were crosswinds* or *a storm that pushed us up higher up above the clouds.*

And then back to the bedside. Emptying the negative pressure reservoir of the exudate, knowing that each cupful contained too much lost protein and that soon the body would begin to feed on itself again, so hurry pilots, find friendly tailwinds. Watching. Watching for eight hours, a quiet shift change to allow rest, but always someone watching, pulse beat by pulse beat. The CCAST weren't asked to heal their patients but to hold them where they were when they were handed over, no worse when they landed, and sometimes, because it had been eight good hours without take-backs to surgery, even a little better.

*

But CCAST hadn't always been there. Thirty years earlier another of Britain's small wars was fought far away. The battle for the Falkland Islands, in the South Atlantic, lasted seventy-four days and was a military victory, despite shortcomings in every aspect of the operation. Supply lines were so strained that by the time the victorious British army arrived in the capital of Port Stanley, they were starving, and for the first time in nearly a century there was looting by troops for basic food and water.[9] Medical provision for the 255 casualties was, despite the efforts of regimental medical officers and surgeons, basic. Everything was the opposite of Afghanistan, and nowhere could this be seen more clearly than in the case of a young Scots Guardsman, Robert Lawrence, who fought and fell on Tumbledown Mountain on the night of 13 June 1982.

Lawrence was part of a mission to take a high ground position, from where the capital would be encircled and the enemy defeated. Initially it was successful, then everything went wrong. The enemy was waiting for them, and there was heavy shelling, snipers and hand-to-hand fighting across impossible terrain in terrible weather – 40 knot winds and blizzards, freezing temperatures. There was no protection against the weather, let alone the weapons of the enemy – a woollen beret instead of a helmet, and no body armour. Lawrence had been on the mountain for several hours and his battalion were beginning to make progress when he was shot in the head by a high-velocity bullet that blew away half his brain, bringing him crashing to the ground. He could feel the wound it left behind, hot and searingly painful, so he thought he would pack it with the snow that lay on the ground around him, which was when he found he couldn't move. And in the meantime, blood – not enough to kill him there and then but bad enough.

There were helicopters to evacuate casualties off the mountain, but not enough of them, and they were only a means of transport, nothing else. Broken radios and general chaos meant it took two and a half hours for one to get there, and when they loaded him up, there wasn't really enough room in the cabin so 'his head ended up hanging out of the door as they flew along.'[10] At the field hospital no one thought he would make it, so he went to the back of the queue for surgery. But he did survive, and after four hours his head was operated on to clear away the dead brain tissue and bullet fragments. Then he was taken to a hospital ship moored in the bay. No pain relief because it was thought to mask symptoms. He had a nine-inch-long wound that began above his right eye and disappeared over the top of his head, constant, thrumming pain and nightmares – dreadful nightmares, for which the answer was a coffee or a beer and a cigarette with whoever had the night shift. Then to Uruguay for an excruciatingly painful brain scan that made the ever-present pain even worse. But the scan confirmed he could fly home for treatment safely, on a VC10, which could hold sixty-eight stretchers in three tiers up and down its metal sides, with aircrew – stewards not medics – who walked up and down a central aisle to mind their passengers (they were never really patients) during the seventeen-hour flight.

Lawrence's injuries had left him partially paralysed on his left side, with a flailing arm that hung down the side of his body. He had some initial physio on the hospital ship and was coming to understand somehow that this would probably be permanent, but the pain was all that filled his head now, so he took a bottom bunk, because he could get into it and picked his own arm up when it dropped out of the cot on to the floor. He could only tell it had fallen out by looking over to see, and the steward walking by kept treading on the arm without him realising. At one point he was brought a meal, a proper old-school aircraft meal, with portions of stuff in separate little plastic compartments. He was handed it as he lay in his place and then left alone. He was incapable of eating it where he was, but he worked out that he could manage it if he got out and sat on the floor, leaning up against the cot. Hunched over the meal, he scooped out the food with a plastic fork in his one good hand.[11] One of the plastic compartments had some black goo-like sauce in it, and he was about to try it to see what it was when he realised that it had come from him – blood and cerebral fluid oozing out of the wound on his head, pooling on the tray. There had been air trapped in his head wound, enough to be affected by the change in cabin pressure, and it had caused the leak. And the pressurisation had made his pain worse, but it was so bad by now that worse meant nothing very much overall. Around him the others on the aircraft assumed he would die at some point during the journey or at least soon afterwards, but Lawrence held on, alone and untended, and willed himself home.

Lawrence survived more brain surgery and sub-standard rehabilitation and today lives with the paralysis and the pain from his injury thirty years before (he calls his useless arm 'Elliot the watchholder'). His memoir of his wounding and of the deficient military response to it, *When the Fighting Is Over: Tumbledown, A Personal Story*, was considered hugely controversial when it was written in 1988, but he was right, and it only got worse. Deficiency in the Defence Medical Service became outright degradation after years of spending cuts. In 1997 the House of Commons Defence Committee questioned whether the Defence Medical Service could actually survive, given that they were 'not sufficient to provide proper support to the front line [...] and show little prospect of being able to do so in the future'.[12] If there is no available military medical service, then a nation cannot go to war. An entire service, not just a hospital, Gone Black.

So it changed. Proper funding, a new strategic plan and the intention of providing something close to NHS-standard care delivered, ten years later, the system described in this book. The men and women who made it happen are still in the service (so still no names), still making improvements to the system – marginal gains now – refining well past their original targets and one day, hopefully, preparing to write their own books telling of their work. How self-aid, buddy aid, team medics, combat medical technicians, MERT, Bastion and the flight home on CCAST became the best system for managing severe casualty from the point of wounding in military medical history. In 2009 another committee could report that care of the wounded serviceman was exemplary, with much to teach the NHS in terms of trauma provision.[13]

*

Two patient memoirs – Lawrence's *When the Fighting Is Over* and Ormrod's *Man Down* – thirty years and an entire world of casualty provision apart. As I wrote about the best, I wanted to remember the worst. And no matter how good the system gets, being wounded is the same. Across the years, a human falls, in paralysis and pain, a new life from that moment on, high-velocity rifle bullet or IED. Mark Ormrod was the first triple amputee to be brought home with his own medical team, on a Tristar aircraft that made multiple stops for refuelling and wasn't quite yet the expert space of the Globemaster. He lay in one of three medical beds in what would otherwise be the first-class cabin. There were actual passengers (officers) returning from deployment just feet away, and no privacy curtains. For hour after hour they could do nothing but watch as the medical team tended the patient and their lifelines, as the injury bit deep, muscles wasting, skin tone fading, all straps and flesh ending where it shouldn't. And sometimes these passengers knew that there were coffins being transported to the rear as well and that, no matter how their tour had gone, it had come down to this journey, across the continents, the barely living alongside them, the dead at the back.[14]

*

Back to the clatter and watchfulness of the Globemaster, flying all the way home, without stopping. There was a hard thump as the wheels dropped ready for landing. One nurse always remembered two things from her CCAST service: dragging the vacuum mattress out of the plane to wash it after the patient was gone, and the impact of that sound. On leave she avoided her local post office because it had an old-fashioned franking machine, and its heavy chunk down on the envelopes reminded her of the punch-thump of the wheels and the work she did high above the earth, securing her leg of the journey back, and what it asked of her in the unceasing rattle and hum.[15]

Landing, deplaning, transferring lines and tubes and batteries, one ambulance per patient non-negotiable, paperwork. Then a new, different, demanding responsibility after every carry, even those where they had been on duty for forty hours straight, including the immersive intensity of the flight. The nurse team leader went all the way to the ward with the patient to see their families. A short conversation, holding themselves straight, even breaths, a last effort to keep the strain off their faces as they quietly explained what they had already written in the patient diary, that *the flight was smooth,* that maybe *there was a bit of a wobble, but they were always watching.* And they gave them the actual diary: *Here, you can read it yourself, later or when you have time, please do, it will help you understand that your loved one was never alone, not for a minute. There's a map that shows where we were flying when you were getting to Birmingham, resolving to be brave no matter what or at least to stop crying, waiting for us to land, hearing the blue-light police escort for our ambulance, fearing the meaning of the sound of sirens.* A handover to the Critical Care staff at Birmingham and then over.

The medical handover to the Critical Care staff in Birmingham wasn't quite the end of their mission. The last thing was the journey back to wherever their aircraft was homed. Before Globemasters this was Lynham, a two-hour drive from Birmingham that felt like four when every last one of their resources was gone (easier once they moved to Brize Norton, which was only an hour away). The aircraft would be waiting, so they went back up inside to clean up. They threw away the absorbent sheets, washed the mattress, stowed the equipment and set it recharging, so it would be ready for the next team. Then, whatever lay ahead, a twenty-four-hour break, and in the meantime another team came on duty at Brize, ready in two hours, and waited for the Globemaster to collect them, where they wait now, today, as you are reading this, in case they are needed, as they were in Tunisia, in June 2015, bringing the wounded back home from the attacks on the beaches.

For the Afghan cohort, CCAST did it all in one day, came home, short break, and the next day went out again, back across the continent, high in the sky to collect another patient. Freight clipped in where the stretcher would go, and unofficially a bit of light smuggling: after all, it was a very large aircraft, and what else were nooks and crannies for if not for fresh food, always at a premium at Bastion. Fruit – one anaesthetic consultant brought a pineapple with him so regularly that anyone seeing it knew that he was on the CCAST that shift. Fruit and milk. Especially milk – fresh milk for brews was currency in the desert, where one could dream of bowls of cereal in good cold milk. Cornflakes in UHT weren't wonderful, so they were mostly used with chocolate melted in the microwave for crispie birthday cakes.

On one flight a nurse decided to borrow the night-vision goggles and look out of the windows at the darkness they moved through. As she remembered what she saw, she suddenly looked past me, back into a different distance. She told of how the Globemaster doesn't have a lot of windows, and after a few minutes she decided that was a good thing, because actually she didn't really need to be reminded that there was so much sky, so many stars, that's really all there was out there, for hours and hours, and suddenly, against the infinity, the aircraft didn't seem master of anything, just a small, grey shape, holding itself, holding everyone in it, ploughing through the darkness and clouds, bringing them home.

PART TWO

HOME

'What happened when I got home?'

12

Birmingham

GATHERING. While the aircraft is in the air, other messages are going out to the next of kin of the injured soldier. The staff in the casualty's regiments reach for the records that tell them names and addresses of the families whose lives have changed at the same moment without feeling the heartbeat under the soil or the dust settling. Contact, this the most dreaded of all messages, no easier with speed and emails and smartphones than it was a century ago, when streets' worth of families with soldiers at the Western Front dreaded the arrival of the postman and the slow walk up to their door. By 1918 one mother could no longer stand even the sight of a letter, so her husband had their post delivered to their neighbour, every piece of it, and she checked it carefully and then put a geranium in a pot on her kitchen window sill to indicate that it was safe for him to come and collect and read out the letters from their son that meant he lived still.[1] In the twenty-first century 'kin' is a more fluid term than previously. Family members, loved ones, previously loved ones, loved ones who can barely stand to be in the same room as the others – all the complications temporarily swept away by the sudden presence in a drive, on a doorstep, of someone who has somehow always been there but only today become solid and breathing, hand out, introducing themselves.

As the casualty notification officers ask if they might come inside to talk, time, in the lives of the family, gains an extra second, like a leap year, but one that will always be a part of their chronometry. The second before they know, the second when life is normal and ongoing and where they could decide to close the door and not hear the words ever, the second every morning just as they wake before they remember and it all comes crashing down.[2] Suddenly, everything becomes very formal, as they are asked by someone they may know well, who is wearing the regimental tie that is suddenly not a welcome sight, who knows perfectly who they are, if they are the person named on the Next of Kin form as the first person to be told. Sometimes, often, when they are asked 'Are you …?' they say NO. No, I am not that person. They try to get back to the second before, blink and wake up, but they are asked again and somehow they move inside the building, and then next comes the news, of injury, its severity, or of death. A second officer then joins them, usually from a car waiting outside, and the practical necessities begin.

The heartbeat under the soil, rippling out, round and further, dust settling and then blowing up again in sudden, blinding gusts. Other phones ring, siblings, exes, best friends. Deciding who to ring first, finding they are out, trying again and again. Allocating the job of notification within the family group to those beyond – someone has to ring them, and the others and then more others, and if they aren't there, find someone who can tell them. Find them today. Minimise will only hold so long at Bastion, and then the news starts to leak out to comrades and families. The military sends out text messages to advise of casualty or loss to the whole battalion. It will be on the news. Mobile phones are wonderful things except when the signal is patchy, as it was for Mark Ormrod's girlfriend, who was told by his twin sister standing out in a cold garden trying to find a signal on Christmas Eve.[3] Sometimes the message coming through is patchy in other ways: Mark's family were told that he had lost one leg when it was actually two, and an arm.

Telling of death is simpler and yet infinitely harder than

telling of injury. What will happen after a death is the same every time, and it will be days before those told are reunited with those gone, standing in the family room at the same RAF station at Brize Norton where the CCAST team wait, while a coffin is unclipped from the stanchions on the Globemaster and slowly brought down to the ground, ordered step by ordered step, in time.

Injury is more complicated. So the casualty notification officers keep it simple. *The loved one is very badly injured, but strong enough to move, they will need a great deal of treatment, including surgery and all the details will be explained to you when you get to Birmingham, so you need to gather up yourselves and whoever else you need with you and get there and by then they can tell you everything. And this is when you should aim to get to Birmingham, as close to the arrival of their loved one as possible so there isn't too much waiting around.* Birmingham, as all military families know by now, means the Queen Elizabeth Hospital in Edgbaston, which contains the designated ward and Critical Care facility for military patients and, unsurprisingly, specialises in trauma and orthopaedics. The main military ward used to be at Selly Oak, not far from Edgbaston, but unexpected survivors needed more than the facilities of a hospital that had treated casualties going back a century to Passchendaele in 1917. So the ward was moved inside the brand-new university hospital (although to keep it simple, from now on I'll use the term 'Birmingham' to cover both).

So they get themselves to Birmingham, phones ringing all the way, and meet in the car park. Sometimes as they wait for everyone to get there, they hear the police sirens that escort every ambulance carrying a casualty to the hospital, and then they see another group across the car park, gathering together, waiting, same red eyes and staggered steps as if at any moment the earth would crumble under their feet, and they don't want to go in with them, because this other loved one is sure to be worse off, closer to death, less recognisable. And then what do they say in the lift up to wherever it is they are both going?

What will they say – how will they even be supposed to look the first time they see their own loved one? Other people parking their cars, with ordinary appointments for ordinary conditions in ordinary lives, see them gathered in their tight tangle of arms wrapped around each other, and look up from their appointment letters with the directions to consultants' rooms and halfway up the stairs realise why the knots of people are there.

*

And all the while, in the ambulance, patient and CCAST travel along a carefully planned route into the city, police getting them through the Birmingham traffic as fast as possible, because they could hold the casualty steady for only so long at the end of this journey. Cars, motorbikes, even mountain bikes, who moved around them, and held back lines of traffic so they could pass, evenly, without stopping, with sirens in the background while the CCAST nurse sat with the patient and thought about the conversations to come. Then unloaded and into a separate entrance from the public ones at the hospital. Elsewhere in the building others gathered to wait for the patient in the ambulance with the police siren escort. Much earlier in the day came a signal from Bastion, a bleep to the on-call trauma registrar, and a MIST report – very basic information:

Mechanism of injury
Injury sustained
Symptoms and vital signs
Time of wounding.

The junior trauma surgeon who had been at Bastion had been promoted and had become a military trauma registrar. It was his bleep that went off, just after the 9-Liner was received, and even though he was driving in to Edgbaston, a little bit of him always went back there into the desert, waiting in a trauma bay, knowing what was about to be rushed from the Chinook into his hands. But at home his job was different. Because of his experience in Bastion, he knew what every element of the MIST report meant, and so he could summon exactly the right team – whoever he wanted for the injury on its way to them. The military trauma registrar had the power to get the most senior consultants in the country out of bed, into scrubs and ready to work. They came to The Bunker – a very basic room, not really very bunkerish. Whiteboards populated the walls, and the military trauma registrar started to write on these with the patient's information, but he didn't need to write much because they all knew what was coming. Then they started planning what would be definitive repair – hopefully, the repair that would stand the new human being in good stead for the rest of their life. A line was drawn and held by MERT and at Bastion, but at Birmingham patients were in Critical Care for weeks and months, not just twenty-four hours. For multiple surgeries. Back and forth, in and out, again and again, 'where multiple trips to theatre should not be seen as failure but as providing a high standard of evidenced-based care'.[4]

And while the men and women in The Bunker planned the restoration, the patient moved from the ambulance, up in the lifts, on to the Critical Care unit. Lines and tubes, take care, just like CCAST, and the next thing, simple: a wash. Their flight was long, and even though the CCAST nurses did their best to keep their exposed skin cool and clean on board the flight, they got hot and sweaty and had to be peeled off the mattress when they arrived. So, before they were put in a proper bed, with sheets and pillows, they were gently cleaned, and their eyes were wiped, and chapped lips tended too, and teeth brushed, with a toothbrush and toothpaste.[5] Made fresh, so they looked like their old selves, sort of, some of them tanned by the Afghan sun, flip-flop marks on their feet, if they had feet, still recognisable and without the smells and dust of their journey and their suffering hanging about them. Gently into bed, lines changed and checked, the first of so many tests, stumps elevated and supported with specially shaped pillows, sheets carefully replaced, and one of those little round dough-nut pillows under their head, so they didn't get occipital alopecia. (It was common, nevertheless, and became known as the Headley Halo after the Headley Court rehabilitation centre – not dangerous but really upsetting once people are strong enough to see themselves in a mirror.) And then every hour or so, until the patient could do this on their own, move-ment, rolling, even if it took four or five people, so that their skin wasn't broken down under the weight of their broken body to form bed sores. And when the first set of tests came back, into theatre, prepped and waiting for them since the first bleep and MIST report, for the first dressing change, definitive repair hopefully beginning.

13

The Duty Critical Care Nurse

The main thing is not to get it wrong; if you
get things wrong, it's all lost.

Duty Critical Care Nurse, Birmingham, 2010

IN A SMALL PALE PINK ROOM on the fourth floor of the hospital
the CCAST crew member met the families and did their best
to explain the journey that had got them all to this point, from
Afghanistan to here, to this room in Birmingham off a corridor
that led to the Critical Care unit, where their loved one lay. *It's
all in there, in the diary, there was a bit of a wobble three or four
hours ago but we took care of it, of him, and we got here safely.
And I'll say goodbye now and wish you all good luck, the next few
months won't be easy but he's a tough, brave lad, and I'll hand you
over to someone who can answer all your questions.*

And then from the background came a nurse, with a white
tunic on, and she thanked the CCAST member and introduced herself with her name and her title. She was the Duty
Critical Care Nurse (DCCN), and from then on, she said, for
the next few most difficult days while their loved one was still
unconscious, they should come to her with whatever questions
they might have: she was easy to spot (that's why she'd got the
white tunic, to make her stand out from all the other nurses
who went past them in blue) and she was there for them.

By 2010 casualty numbers from Afghanistan pressed in on

the staff at Birmingham. And even though they had moved into a bright, shiny, new hospital with more beds and a bigger lift, there were too many family groups arriving at once, too much to tell them, too many people to liaise with. So things went wrong, or went slowly, information muddled or late; it deepened suffering in a place where it lapped up the walls anyway.[1] So a new nursing role was created – unique in the profession, unique to Birmingham: the Duty Critical Care Nurse, who did nothing else but care for the families and make sure she never got anything wrong. Her first day on the job was the first ever after the job was created, and saw the most ever casualties admitted at once to Birmingham, and the most ever families arriving to see them.

The first person on the job could and did cope. They had made a really good choice: just the right combination of strength, clear thinking and compassion. I can vouch for it because I interviewed her, and I felt better just walking into her office (although I had to explain to her that she didn't have to keep her military hat on while she talked to me, because she hadn't been sure of the protocol for historians).

She'd nursed in the field hospital in Iraq, where the wind blew sand into every nook as she worked, and the mortars rained down, crash crash crash every day, where she slept in a concrete pod known as a coffin for safety and where she reckoned there was a good chance that she would come home in an actual one, alone in the back of the aircraft. Then to Afghanistan. At Bastion there was no more fear, and an experience she cherished: being part of the team in the trauma bays and wards that provided the second and last lines of defence against death, and sent more men home alive than had ever been done before. She wrote patient diaries for the men she saw off to the CCAST team, to share how they had worked together for their survival. She wrote patient diaries for the families of men who died in her ward, so their families would know of their last hours.

Then to Birmingham, where her job was to care for the

families she had written for in patient diaries, the people she had only imagined as she wrote, seeking to find ways to make the worst thing in the world a little bit easier. Watching the group, reading the room, face by face, to see who is the natural leader, who she should speak to – a mum, or a dad, or a sibling, or the patient's other half, whoever has moved themselves most quickly to her side, is paying closest attention, not lost in crying. Sometimes – rarely, but sometimes – she could not read the room. The faces were tear-stained, shocked and hostile. A mum who repeated over and over that her son needed to go home now. A dad whose rage at his son's wounding exploded from him over her and everyone there, and it took a good two or three days of clear speaking and careful silences before the situation turned and he came to trust her. Then the broken families, two families, learning the technique of getting them on either side of the patient's bed, mothers of children, current partners, complicated, trust, clarity, getting it right.

She pushed open the door from the pale pink room to the grey-blue corridor and led them out, moving resolutely, making sure they were all coming with her, the questions starting now, the space changing as they moved – the pale pink room was utterly foreign, but in the ward was their family member, so the space they occupied was somehow theirs too. The first sight would be the hardest of all, she knew, because nothing could quite prepare them for that room, where all the patients – everyone someone's child – were almost disappeared under their tubes and machines, broken into unidentifiable pieces, thin, bloodshot, eyes swollen into dark blue slits, skin ashen. Part of her job was guiding them up to the bedside, standing at one end, introducing them to the nurses in their blue tunics with the long plastic aprons and disposable gloves, who have momentarily stopped their work and who nod their greeting and then turn back to the patient. They may have been given aprons and gloves before they could move slowly closer and closer, daring to touch, softly speaking the patient's name, checking that he really can't hear them, murmuring, crying again. They saw the human, underneath the tubes, saw that he is still big enough to fill a bed, and then there are the parts of their human they don't recognise – heavily bandaged stumps and limbs, swollen bigger than a boxing glove, that lay where hands should lie. And this is not a dream, they are not waking up; this is how it will be from now on.[2]

The other nurses or the consultants or the professors started to explain what was happening and what was going to happen. The DCCN listened as intently as the family because they wouldn't remember everything that was said or understand it, and it was her job to remind them. They needed all the help they could get to become used to this new place in their lives, with the machines in it beeping and flashing, and they did so quite quickly: a bed is a bed, after all, sheets and blankets, even with all the tubes, head raised slightly on a pillow because that really helped them not to get ventilator-associated pneumonia.[3] Sometimes the DCCN saw those at the end of the bed surreptitiously patting down the sheets to feel where the limbs ended, even peeping under the sheets to see where the tubes and lines went and if what was left was recognisable ('Mum, you're going to be taller than me again', one amputee patient would say after waking to his mother).[4]

Then, after all of it, she guided them back down the corridors, into the lift and back to the car park for the drive home. In a way it was easier if the patient hadn't been awake enough to see their reactions when they looked down at what was left of him. One patient understood this much later, when he saw the pain flicker back across the faces of his family several weeks after he came back home, and he was grateful he hadn't been awake that day to see it for the very first time.

*

There is a scale for sedation – the Richmond scale – and the ideal is 0 (zero), for 'Alert and Calm'.

The Richmond Scale

−1	Drowsy	Not fully alert; sustained awakening to a voice that says their name; some eye opening/ eye contact for up to ten seconds
−2	Light sedation	Briefly awakens with eye contact to voice for less than ten seconds
−3	Moderate	Movement or eye opening to voice but no eye contact
−4	Deep sedation	No response to voice but movement or eye opening to physical stimulus, usually by gently shaking their shoulder or rubbing their chest
−5	Unarousable	No response to voice or physical stimulus

Waking is almost never as simple as feeling a touch and hearing a voice say your name. Sedatives are withdrawn slowly, a little every day, under careful supervision from the anaesthetist.[5] Then as they go from a −4 to −3 up to −1, things can and usually do start to unravel. Almost everyone, soldiers and civilians alike, who wakes on a Critical Care ward finds the aftermath really difficult: altered agitated mental states, problematic memory, a very odd environment. Patients can't understand why they are there, what is being done to them, and they lash out, yanking on tubes and lines, ripping them out: 'the literature contains multiple reports of fatal self-extubations and removal of intravascular devices.'[6] So there are usually restraints discreetly nearby, pharmacological or actual, hand mitts or soft straps for limbs on bed rails, and these are applied and monitored continually until the storm passes.

Waking soldier-casualties was worst of all, because they also had to contend with a collision of two worlds: Afghanistan and home. The storm began in Afghanistan, blinding sunlight, fighting, explosions, pain, those gathered around them shouting, shouting, then blackness. In the blackness they travelled thousands of miles, across continents, time passing pulse beat by pulse beat for the CCAST crew but stopped for them, and when they woke, it resumed, hearing first, slamming them back in the fire fight, still fighting, still on the ground in the dust, the enemy about them, and they scream for help, except the light in the blue-grey ward is dimmer, and the group gathered around them spoke softly, no more shouting.[7] And no matter what anyone could tell them, their brain assumed capture, that the huge room with the inhuman light was a torture chamber, the lines in their arms and legs full of poison, the catheter in their bladder a bomb, and pain was rushing in so it must be true; the men and women around them were masked, covered in plastic, with unnatural hands in blue gloves, so torturers, interrogators – don't listen to the words that come from behind the masks trying to soothe them.[8] And their families were there, in Afghanistan, where there was nothing but danger, nothing, danger and pain, and whoever else was there they must get their families OUT of Afghanistan, OUT NOW. So the families were got away, just to the corridor, and the figures in blue swarmed over their patient and quietened him again, from the shouting and the wrenching.

So there is another component to the Richmond Scale: the Agitation Scale.

+4	Combative	Overly combative, violent, immediate danger to staff
+3	Very agitated	Pulls or removes tubes or catheters, aggressive
+2	Agitated	Frequent non-purposeful movement, fights ventilator
+1	Restless	Anxious but movements not aggressive or vigorous

Gradually, moving back down the scale, patients had longer periods awake, and the fragments from the war that burst out – call signs, orders to get down, swearing – dissolved and were replaced by ordinary hallucinations from the medications

– forklift trucks driving up and down the ward, strange creatures in the room with them, distortions of the faces of their visitors. They are awake enough by now to have the process explained to them, so somewhere in the very back of their mind there is enough understanding of their situation to keep them calm in the swirl. Families and the DCCN show them their patient diaries – going through the entries with them, hour by hour, showing them how they were carried by MERT, and CCAST, kept alive in the Bastion Critical Care unit and visited by their friends, who wrote messages for them, in their new future. Filling in the gaps. Every name, every entry, sparked a connection, memories, pulse beats, time evening itself out, two worlds becoming one new one. Days became days, and nights became nights. Eventually, the families didn't need the diary any more and they could leave it at home (Scott Meenagh remembered his mother thought the diary was the most wonderful thing to have while she watched him before he woke), because everyone in or gathered around the bed understood where they were and was preparing for the next stage of the journey.

The next stage is breathing on their own. Most of the patients in Birmingham will have been intubated to help them breathe. Taking the breathing tube out – extubating – is the very last step in the process. A machine will keep them alive, but it cannot do enough to make them live. And the longer they are on the machine that breathes for them, the more dangerous it is. The muscles that inhale and exhale start to weaken, and the sort of gunk that is normally coughed away builds up; and gunk is an excellent breeding ground for infection, pneumonia, worsening respiratory failure – more machine, less person, less life. So eventually the tube for the ventilator that was so skilfully and carefully inserted back on the Chinook by the MERT had to be removed, and the breathing last done unassisted on the ground in Afghanistan had to resume.

Preparing for extubation takes a long time and is complicated. It can begin only when the patient is sufficiently clear of infection that they can be touched without the plastic gloves and aprons and masks in between, because touch – human to human, contact practice – is the only way it works. So meet the physiotherapist. Physiotherapists are primary contact practitioners; physiotherapy is defined as the treatment of disease, injury, or deformity by physical methods such as massage, heat treatment and exercise rather than by drugs or surgery. Even though most of us think of bad backs or sports injury when we think of physios, we are just as likely to see them working on trauma patients, especially orthopaedic trauma, in Critical Care wards. Increasingly, whether military or civilian, physios are seen as an essential part of the multi-disciplinary team, preventing Critical Care patients getting worse by just lying there. The families on the military ward at Birmingham know all about this now as they've been watching physios work on the ward, in other bed spaces, since they came in.[9]

It is physios, they realise, who are carefully rolling or moving patients who are not yet awake. Rolling a patient on to their side increases the volume of the uppermost lung, and increased volume means a better-functioning lung. And while they are on their side, gently tilting the neck so that the head faces downward helps to clear gunk. Roll and tilt, return, roll and tilt: ventilated lungs work better and clearer, extra oxygen is absorbed more easily, everything closer to normal rather than further away. Roll and tilt and return. Gentle chest massage also keeps gunk production down, and improves circulation. Gentle joint massage, where there still are joints, does the same thing, stimulating circulation, slowing muscle wastage, all of which needs to begin to work properly when the patient can breathe again. Physios work quietly at the bedside, learning their patient, learning their sounds and the feel and temperature of their skin, moving them slowly across this part of the landscape, as softly as a palm placed in the small of a back to guide them up to a door.

Getting the patient ready to breathe on their own is called 'weaning'. It can never come too quickly for the family, because fewer machines means recovery going the right way, but the

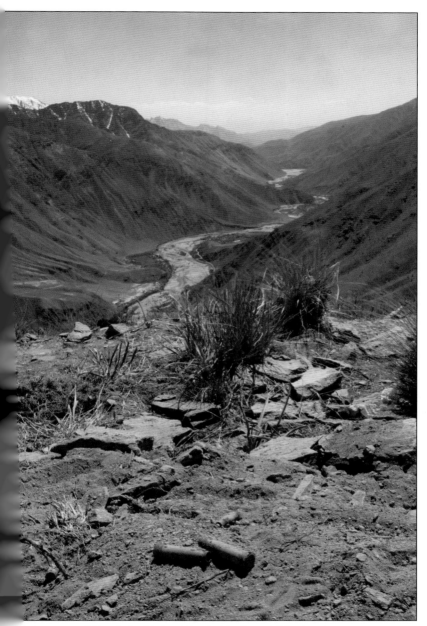

Historic fortified position in Northern Afghanistan.

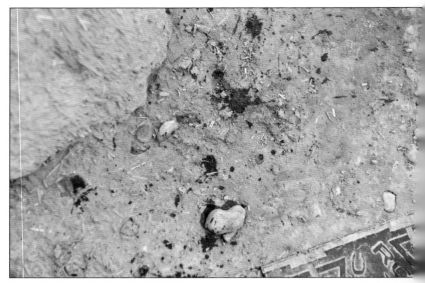

Afterwards, IED.

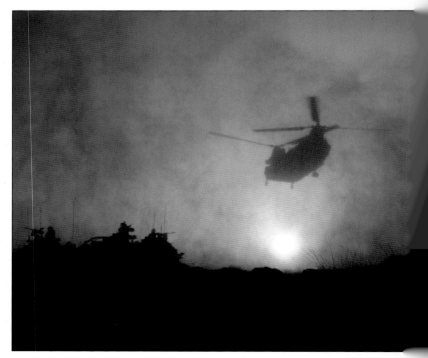

Securing a landing site for the Chinook.

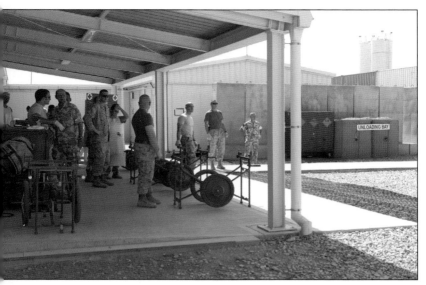

Waiting for MERT to land, outside Field Hospital Camp Bastion.

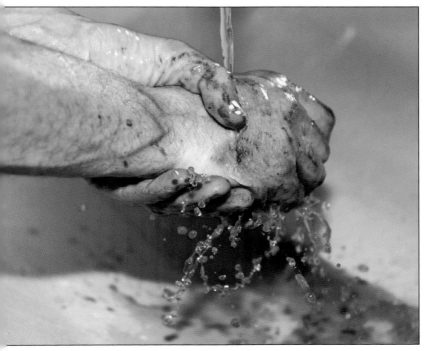

Afterwards, sink near trauma bays, Bastion.

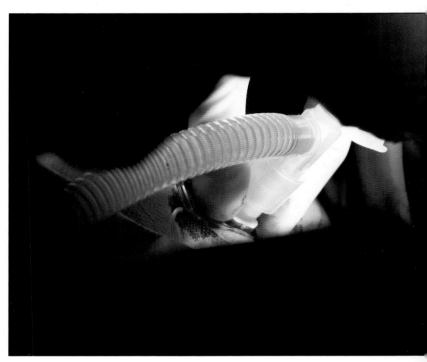

Intubation.

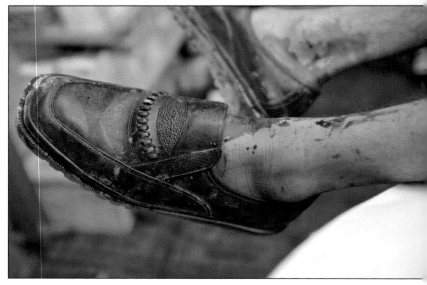

Eighty per cent of the hospital's patients were locals.

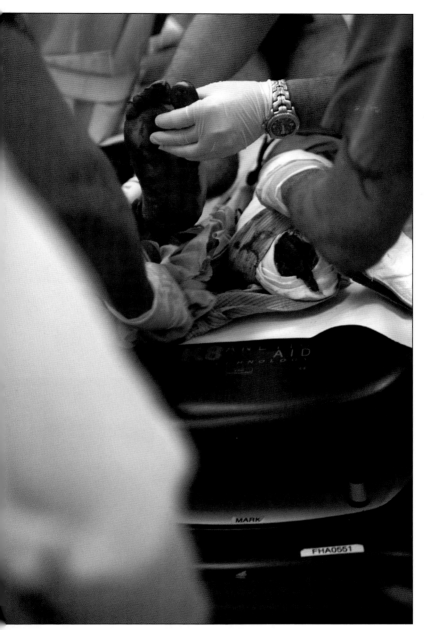

Traumatic amputation with avulsive soft tissue injuries.

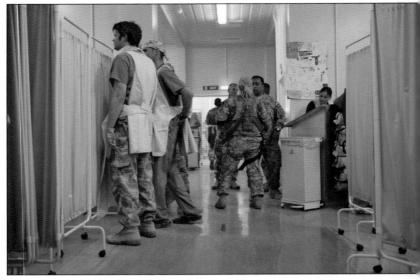

Watching Trauma Bay 7, Bastion.

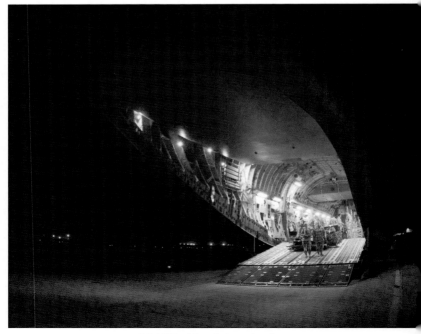

CCAST taking their patient home.

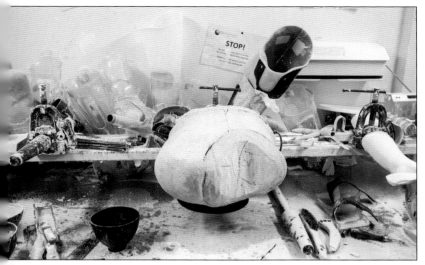

Hard-plug replica of an amputation stump in the prosthetists' workshop at Headley.

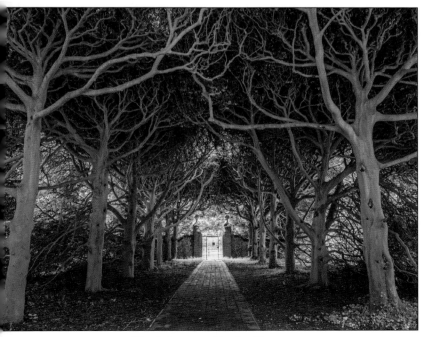

The Arboretum, Headley Court.

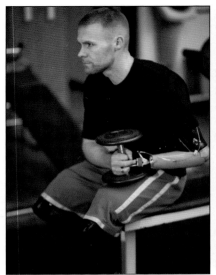

Mark Ormrod.

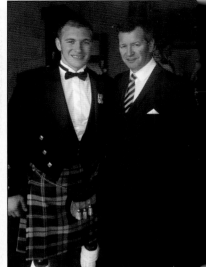

Scott Meenagh, Thomas Meenagh.

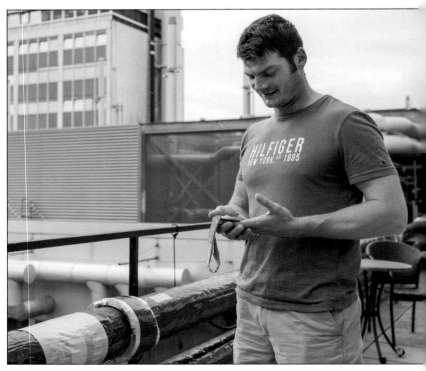

Dave Henson at Imperial College London with his Paralympic medal, 26 September, 2016

patient is often not so sure. Anxious, used to the ventilator, dependent, worried what will happen when it stops, suffocating – maybe we should just leave it for the time being and see where we get to. In the end it is the physios who do respiratory work who are the experts on the use of ventilators. They will be mobilising their patients now, mobilising, like with troops, calling up their muscles, step by step, even if they are still a little sedated. They need to get their lungs working, their respiratory muscles, like all their other muscles, devastated by the injury and its aftermath, back to something near functional. They'll need to learn to cough again, and to cough they need to sit up – and they can see in the eyes of the patient that they think that seems about as likely as asking them to fly across the room. But, even if it takes four physios together to raise the patient gently in the bed, saying *don't worry about the tubes and lines, we've got those,* suddenly they are sitting up, swinging whatever legs the patient has over the side of the bed, head up, for the first time since going down, looking around at where they are.

The physio helps with the movements to start with, but eventually leaves the patient to do it on their own. And just sitting up helps with core, and balance, even without really trying. Every moment spent upright is medical pure gold – no drugs, no machines – just one human being expertly guiding another into a new space. Even ventilated oxygen distributes itself better as the patient moves, and that will mean better circulation, better digestion, the body getting going again. It helps with the hallucinations too, and the space between sedations gets longer and calmer and more work can be done.[10]

More physio over the next day and week. The cough is vital, so the muscles that do the coughing must be continually worked and strengthened. Stand up, sit up, raise their arms up and down, breathe in and out to increasingly longer counts – hold their breath for a few counts, relaxed breath out, huffing (almost as important as coughing). The physio tries to get the patient to be able to do things on their own – cough, huff, sit, lift themselves, roll to the side. For patients with multiple amputations this is sometimes too demanding, so the physio is there at their side, at their joints, gently massaging to restore circulation and prevent contraction by the new scars, which cover their bodies like paint splatters. For those patients without a knee joint, the best exercise is to get them to roll over completely, on their front, and then carefully lift the stump a little backwards, and then a little more, making what muscles are left remember what work is like. Strong and long hip flexor muscles, in particular, really help when the time comes for a new leg. So everyone came to welcome the work of the physio, because when they said so, up came the prosthetists for a look and the promise of a first prosthetic.

Physios, talking about new legs going in where the space in the bed is, meant more to the patients than any other conversation they had since they arrived in Birmingham. It meant they could see where they were, orientation, interacting with other humans, following instructions, achieving a result, taking back a little control, no longer just someone to whom things were done. A partnership began that would last well beyond Birmingham – and a different kind of conversation, with someone who didn't know what they were like before the deal was done. And beyond the military ward these relationships prove the case for the presence of physios beside all Critical Care beds, part of the early assessment process for civilians of whatever age and diagnosis. There's no magic drug or surgery that gets Critical Care patients moving better than one-to-one physiotherapy. A study across the whole hospital at Birmingham found that physios reduced the stay in Critical Care wards by eight days, with better outcomes both physically and psychologically.[11]

*

One of the physios who courteously but firmly drove this system forward had also been to Afghanistan. He's still in the military, so I still can't tell you his name, but from now on whenever I talk about 'the physio', it's him. He deployed to Camp Bastion twice: the second time between April and September, the hottest time of all, 54 degrees outside. But he wasn't outside much, just moving between the physio tent and the hospital. His presence was part of the principle of the movement of clinical capability forward in war zones, as far forward as it will go, and physio skills, as we have seen, are essential in the Critical Care wards, wherever they may be and whoever the patients are. Most of his patients left in the beds at Bastion were locals, and he worked with them as he worked at Birmingham, slowly, carefully, rolling and tilting, reminding them how to breathe and how to cough. Sitting up, huffing, slowly mobilising their muscles. He worked with an interpreter at his side to explain what he was saying, and he took the patients who could manage it out for short walks in the early-morning sunshine cool of Bastion, and then back to bed, three weeks, four weeks and finally strong enough to go back to whatever waited for them at home.

He did the same for the CPERS, the Captured PERsons, who also spent weeks in the ward, but surrounded by white wheeled screens and heavily armed guards. The guards watched his every move, every roll and tilt and turn, watched as he and other physios lifted their patients to a seated position, then to a bedside chair and then a short walk. Terps did the talking for him, but from behind one of the screens so as not to be identified later, and occasionally one of the guards would call him over to remind him that if he was going to be lifting a patient into a seated position, it would be a good idea for everyone if he remembered to remove his side-arm. When the CPER patients were ready for a longer walk, there was an elaborate manoeuvre where the screens were rolled into a long white corridor so the CPERS could move outside without seeing or being seen by the locals in the camp. His CPER patients had different injury patterns from everyone else he treated at Bastion. Not much blast injury or amputation. On the battlefield they attacked standing up, facing their target, firing semi-automatic weapons and rockets. They had no body armour, and the middle of their bodies made an easy target, so instead they were usually suffering from wounds to the abdomen. These were always full of infection, and bellies could be swelled to bursting with the gas released by the bacteria, so physiotherapy was crucial to restore circulation, mobilisation and intestinal function – getting their bowels going. So the physio worked and rolled and got used to waiting for the interpreter behind the screen to call out whatever it was he called out. Then one day, when they were recovered enough, the guards would come out from behind the screen and take his patients away, he never knew where.

*

The plastic surgeon who had built the garden at Bastion also worked at Birmingham. He never minded seeing the physio at the bedside of his patients on the military ward because physios had tended to his back and neck after long hours at the operating table. In Afghanistan he got used to reading about the wreckage of blast injury, how it hid death deep inside a human being. So he favoured 'meticulous repeated marginal debridements' to preserve as much tissue and functional potential as possible.[12] He saw most patients in theatre every forty-eight to seventy-two hours until the last scrap of dead or infected tissue was gone, going after the smallest fragments driven high and away from the original wound that were difficult to get at, difficult to dig out, keeping the patient sick from infection. The patients couldn't eat solid food six hours before an operation, so a patient who may have been awake, breathing and only just back eating properly, digestion remembering how to do its job, physiologically restoring, was suddenly hungry again, and the lines were back, and the sedation. That was just the start.

Next came the actual reconstruction. Blast injuries are avulsive – they blow skin off high up the limbs away from the bone end, leaving little for surgeons to work with, so they couldn't simply fold over spare skin and muscle and make an end (this is called primary closure). They needed to take skin and ideally muscle with good healthy blood supply from somewhere else altogether and move it to the wound. This is a flap, a much deeper, more complex slice of tissue than a graft, one with all the mechanisms it needs to survive, vessels, arteries, its own little world. This is where they need the microscopes (which they didn't have in Bastion), to connect up the smallest workings, one by one, sometimes taking a whole day in theatre for just a single movement of whole flesh to wound.

Before they could start, they needed to plan these surgeries. More complicated than it sounds. The trick was to find somewhere with enough viable tissue (the 'donor area'), cut it out and work out where it should go. Not just that. These were flaps for young humans; they needed to stick because they'd be making demands on them for a good long while to come, so the soft tissue they moved from one part to the other had to be robust. They didn't take any muscles for free flaps that were used for core stability and which would be essential to rehab when their patients eventually got there. There are some expendable muscles, like those of the inner thigh, or from along the chest, that might not have been damaged in the explosion, so they used those, preferably in a way that meant they didn't have to turn the patient over and then back during the actual surgery. Lines, tubes, touching, trying not to make something almost infinitely complicated any more difficult.[13] And they didn't do anything at all but plan until the patient was stable – no fevers from infection (still called pyrexias, as they were in the First World War), getting proper nutrition and off any strong meds that control things like blood pressure. If they weren't stable, the flaps failed, the donor area was wasted and the patient went four steps back, not forward at all.

So they didn't rush, although a Critical Care ward that was full of young men waiting to be reconstructed sometimes made that impossible. One patient spent forty-five hours in surgery over two months – not unusual – another seventy-five hours, another thirty-three. Keep going back, no matter how slow the healing, or the infection, keep the family informed. Multiple visits to theatre mean the best possible care.[14] And it's why surgeons and patients who had both been at Birmingham during the war are usually pleased to meet and, when they do, ask each other odd questions like 'I can't remember if I operated on you' or 'Do you think you operated on me?' And it's rare that either of them can ever remember, but for a moment there's a bond, a space in time, with no one else in the room, and they chat about how it was, and they both feel a little better afterwards.

For the plastic surgeon, the longest and the hardest case of all was a patient he had first seen at Bastion, one of the worst cases of blast injury, most of one leg simply pulverised. The damage was so extensive that he had had to perform a hind-quarter amputation – a hemipelvectomy – where all of the leg and half the pelvis is removed – like wrenching out the leg on a plastic doll, except there is nothing wrenching about it; it takes hours to repair the nerves and veins and soft tissue around such a huge wound. Hind-quarter amputations are very rarely done in normal medical practice – usually only for cancers where large tumours have grown in the upper thigh.[15] At Bastion it had been worth the decision to operate – life saved, stabilised, future possible. CCAST kept him stable, and got him back to Birmingham, where he spent a year on the ward, back and forth to theatre. The plastic surgeon came to know him well, and was pleased to see that he was managing a wheelchair, becoming more independent, and on one particularly good day they played ping-pong in one of the recreation rooms. And then suddenly the patient developed complications: stability failing, infection, sepsis, bleeding, oxygenated blood not getting where it should, the cascade unstoppable, no future any more, death. For the surgeon who had fought alongside him it was very hard. But there was that afternoon's clinic and the next day's patients, so on he went. Even after the war was over, and the ward cleared, suddenly there was a new MIST report for patients being transported home by CCAST from the attack on holiday-makers in Tunisia, one of them with fifty separate trauma wounds. Days after their discharge he joined military colleagues at a meeting of international civilian trauma experts to advise them how best to organise their units in the aftermath of the Paris attacks of November 2015.

*

Pain, always pain. The consultant who co-ordinated the treatment of pain from point of wounding onwards summed up the challenge they faced at Birmingham in Critical Care and beyond:

> The population we are dealing with often have complex pain issues. We are also dealing with mechanisms of injury that are not routinely seen except in a few centres around the world. To what extent these various injuries created their own patterns of pain is impossible to quantify.[16]

Unexpected survivors at Birmingham were patients in a great deal of pain. Beyond the military ward consultants thought about post-operative pain, post-amputation pain, inflammation pain, all the other kinds of pain, as separate things, affecting separate patients. But for the military cohort all the kinds of pain that can be imagined, all at once, all in one person, all the time. Every stage of treatment, every different procedure had its own challenges of pain (especially dressing changes), different and yet the same. Pain is a continuum.

Back to fundamental principles, because fundamental principles were almost all they had. Pain is not acceptable. Alleviation of pain is a human right. The first stage in the treatment of pain is asking about pain, asking an individual about pain, not looking at the chart that says what should be happening, what they should be feeling. The pain service at Birmingham was entirely individualised because they had no choice, no chart for what was happening, because that's the way it is with unexpected survivors.

Away from the bedside, an infrastructure had to be created to deal with patterns of pain that were impossible to quantify. It was based on a pain team, unimaginatively named the Military Pain Team. The consultant who led it ensured that, whenever members of the team spoke to each other, or the patient, which they did every day, sometimes more, they spoke the same language. Not easy. Pain resists language – not just because the experience of pain can render the sufferer speechless, whimpering, but because it's an innate human problem that our brains are limited in their ability to describe pain objectively.[17] So pain treatment, of any kind, is based on hard (not very good and not very consistent) questions. We've all been there: how does the pain feel? Is it distracting? What is it on a scale of one to ten? Or ten to one, if one or ten is very painful? What colour is it? If your pain was an animal, what animal would it be? Instead the language the pain team spoke was deliberately simple and clear because they used the system the pain consultant and the team thought was the best: the World Health Organisation's pain 'ladder'. The WHO pain ladder is designed to be used for cancer patients, as part of their global initiative to improve treatment and palliative care for non-communicable diseases, but it is based on the same fundamental principles as the pain pathway that started at point of wounding in Afghanistan: wherever and however possible, there should be freedom from pain. Pain should not prompt pain treatment; pain treatment should block pain before it starts or gets worse. So using the WHO pain ladder system, analgesia is given every three to six hours, not on demand. According to the WHO, this is cheaper and much more effective than waiting for the patient to ask or call or cry out.[18] The ladder has three simple steps which determine how much and what kind of analgesia is given:

First step – no pain at rest, mild on movement

Second step – mild pain at rest, moderate on
    movement
Third step – continuous pain at rest, severe on
    movement.

And it is a dynamic ladder: pain is assessed in relation to what
has gone before. (How is pain now? Is it better than before
or worse that before?) Patients can travel up and down the
ladder as their pain gets worse or better, and it is much easier
for everyone if pain can be described comparatively along
the way. Quickly the pain team discovered that, although the
WHO ladder was the right system for them, it wasn't quite
long enough, so at Birmingham it had a fourth step: severe,
uncontrolled pain.

So, as they hoped it had at point of wounding, pain treatment at Birmingham began with a clear question that the
military pain team's patients could answer because it was about
their own pain and its history, and that was less of a hard question because they designed it to be easier. From that they built
individualised, multi-modal treatment. Another fundamental principle. For the kind of pain that requires a fourth step
on the ladder nothing is ever going to work on its own. Mild
drugs, not opioids, starting with paracetamol and ibuprofen.
Nerve blocks and lots of epidurals. Drugs to treat anxiety about
future pain and futures in general. If the pain 'is not amenable
to a regional technique', use drugs to treat pain at the nerve
site. A double hit is best: opioids that treat pain at the place of
pain and where it registers in the brain, modified release or
immediate effect, as strong as necessary, even if that meant the
hallucinations came back. Hallucinations are better than pain:
intense and unpleasant but better than pain.[19] Whatever the
maximum dosage for all the medications was, you can be sure
the pain team used it for their patients who found themselves
trapped and terrified on step four of the pain ladder until they
came back down.

Eventually, most of them did come down, one step at a

time, sometimes backwards then forwards again, and mostly never quite off the ladder, staying on the first step – mild pain, but better than yesterday. It was pain treatment as conversation, where each listened carefully to the questions of the other because they understood the language being used and it was a good place to start; but also, the pain team hoped, it gave their patients some sense of control or at least participation in their own treatment, because the pain team knew they would need it. Pain would follow them out of Birmingham, into rehab and everything would be easier if they understood their pain, and could express it clearly.

Other conversations too, other hard questions, such as why could a patient feel a limb that was clearly no longer there. It was nurses from the pain team who answered that what they were feeling was called a phantom limb, and it was quite normal that they should feel it because phantom limbs have been known about for centuries. Almost everyone who has an amputation, for whatever reason, gets them. Phantom limbs, as they say in the textbooks, are caused by aberrant inputs from the peripheral nervous system travelling to the brain and back again. They are not about memory of injury; psychological factors do not affect who gets a phantom limb, although eventually the suffering degrades the sufferer at all levels. Phantom limbs hurt: pain just like in the rest of the body that the patient can see, but somehow different. Throbbing, knife-like sensations, burning, pricking, cramping. Or just generally very weird. Phantom limbs feel heat, or cold, or moisture or itching, phantom toes crossing, or pins and needles, or flickering like electric shocks, or cramping, lasting for minutes or hours, unpredictable.

At Birmingham they tried to help. In the case of phantom limbs they put a thick stocking end over the stump, if it was healed enough, so the patient could feel its sides and their brains could adjust. The physio came back and gave them exercises that worked with the phantom sensations rather than fighting them: things like bending down to scratch itching invisible feet. Everyone, patient, pain team and physio, at least felt they were doing something, although there is, thus far, not much evidence that it worked.

Nurses waited at bedsides to answer hard questions as they had always waited. In the First World War it was nurses who sat until their post-operative patients were awake enough to hear the news that their legs were gone or that the darkness was never-ending because they had been made blind. At Birmingham genital injury was one of the worst things to prepare a patient for. It was the first thing they asked on waking, only ever semi-joking. One of Scott Meenagh's unit mates wrote in his diary: 'You alright mate? Your balls are okay and I look forward to seeing you soon.'[20] Unexpected survivors meant more and more of it, harder and harder conversations. Blast injury takes a particularly horrifying form on the pelvis. If the pelvis is fractured, or even if the ligaments that hold it in place are snapped, then the ends lose their rounded shape and destroy everything that they used to neatly encircle. Too high for a tourniquet. Blood vessels run across all joints of a pelvis and the ends of the bones rip them open, arterial bleeds. If the blood vessels aren't torn, then other things are, disastrously. Prostate injury, urethral and bladder injuries, colon and bowel perforation. Avulsive injury means loss of penis and testicles. In the trauma bay surgeons applied a pelvic binder to put back some of the shaping and control around the delicate organs. Then complex repairs, fast, direct suturing, an absolute need for speed because poison was leaking into a system that had no ability left to combat it. But practice meant lives were still saved, triple amputees bundled up in their binders and sent on to CCAST for home. Life now, life undignified and painful thereafter, new terms of the deal. So even if surgeons worked for hours repairing, reconstructing, doing what they could, gone is gone. Hardest of all was to explain to a girlfriend or partner that the plans they didn't even know they had for a family, and the means to make one, were now gone too.

14

Mark Ormrod (3)

MARK ORMROD'S EXTUBATION and his recovery from the acute phase of his care were, he would probably be surprised to hear, considered to be pretty straightforward. The first surviving triple on the ward in Birmingham, he also had a bad burns injury from the heat of the explosions, in addition to the very many rips and tears in what was left of his body from shrapnel. As he became gradually aware of his condition, he worried about his tattoo – a huge abstract pattern that went from the base of his spine and flared out towards his shoulders. His girlfriend had to take a photograph to show him that the tattoo was entirely intact. The photo also showed how little of the rest of him was intact. There were deep gouges along his side, debrided into teardrop shapes by the surgeons, and a nasty-looking set of scabs and scars under his arm running into the dressing over the limb stump. He'd not been aware of the first bouts of surgery, but the family round his bedside were, and the news got worse every time he disappeared from the ward. By now they knew that his left leg was gone as well as his right knee, but, as someone told them, the amputation of the left leg was done through the knee and this was a good thing because if the joint could be saved, then walking was going to be so much easier.

Except that a bone fragment had lodged deep in the thick thigh muscle of his left leg stump and it was infected. Back to theatre. They couldn't remove the fragment and stop the infection with minimal debridement, so they had to cut away the entire portion of muscle. There was no more muscle to support what was left of the left knee joint, so the leg had to be shortened to match by four centimetres, so the joint was gone and Mark was the newest member of an exclusive club: a bilateral (both legs), transfemoral (across the thigh bone) amputee.[1] His left arm was safe, but his right arm, which in its dressings looked intact all the way down to the elbow, was also not healing properly, so back into theatre for shortening, almost up to the shoulder. It was suddenly seeing this arm stump that made him realise what was missing: no forearm – further down – no hand – further down – no fingers. And he cried out, thinking it was a nightmare, that he was asleep, but a nurse came over and explained that he was awake, and what he had lost. In the midst of the hallucinations and pain medication he dozed off again, but then each time he woke, there it was, or wasn't, all over again. And what was left looked horrifying. There was a drainage tube sticking out of a green Brillo-pad-type dressing at the end, and Mark did his best to hide it under the sheets whenever the family came. But they'd sat at his bedside in his acute care phase, and they had seen his struggle back from the edge, so they hardly noticed the dressing and its ugly tubing.

It wasn't surprising that Mark reacted so strongly to seeing that his hand was missing. Think about how often you look down and see your hand: even if only out of the corner of your eye, it's in your line of sight most of the day. Huge areas of the brain are dedicated to controlling hands and processing the sensory information sent to it by the fingers, far more than are used for the feet. These areas activate just when you look at your hands, before you've even thought about using them for something, and they activate whether or not your eyes actually find a hand when they look. Mark was experiencing sensory deprivation: agonising, a shock-scream inside the brain every time the eyes look down and send it information that doesn't make sense. And perhaps there are parts of soldiers' brains that are tied to their hands even more closely than everyone else's. Think about saluting.[2] Everyone thinks they know how to do it, but to do it right is difficult; it takes precision. The hand at the end of the arm describes a wide arc and then a slight wrist swivel so the fingertips hit the eyebrow at just the right place, thumb down. The downward movement to put the arm back in place is much shorter, snapping a line down the front of the body, thumb tucked in. No room for variation; it has to be done properly every time. It's an extraordinarily significant, single, small military act. (Just one of the reasons why the hand surgeon at Bastion fought so hard for every hand he could save.)

For Mark, some good news, finally. He'd had a CT scan of his head, and it showed no traumatic brain injury. The hallucinations were just from the drugs; what everyone could see of him was what he would be from now on, with the same capacity to cope and rebuild. On 2 January Mark finally moved out of Critical Care and into his own room on the Burns and Plastics ward. He was getting to know the plastic surgeons and the physios who were planning his rehabilitation, but most of all he was getting to know his new body, only two-thirds the size it had been before the explosion, and the endless new consequences for his new frame. He was awake for the whole day and trying to sleep at night, something like normal, but it was boiling hot in his room, for no good reason other than useless hospital ventilation, no openable windows as usual, and his body was covered in sweat, on no sleep, hour after hour, night after night, so he was grumpy with his nurses and family. His truncated body tried and failed to cool itself – no soles of feet, no palms of hands, leg surface area mostly gone so no way to vent the heat, but with the same amount of blood pumping round half the area, heat keeps coming. Heat made worse because Mark had multiple burns and new graft sites from the multiple surgeries needed to keep his wounds clean and make viable stumps for him. So the wounds were hot, and the donor sites, where the flaps had come from, were hot and bruised and electrified with pain to the touch.

And he had an infection. The smallest thing on the wards in Birmingham, but by far the most deadly, feared as killers as they had been on the Western Front; we're better at controlling them now, but not perfect. The hectic in the blood.[3] Debridement after debridement and still casualties had contamination blasted deep into their tissues that no one could find or get at. And the surgeons can't take infinite amounts of tissue away, because something has to remain as a bed for grafting, so very broad-spectrum antibiotics are part of the complex of lines running into the patients as they are admitted to Birmingham.

Bacteria run rampant on a human body with uncontrolled tissue damage, weakened by blood loss.[4] They grow on the spot, and then they spread deep inside the human body, infecting the whole system, and they do it fast. They cause a system to go septic – sepsis, dreaded in operating wards. Infections produce toxins, which damage small blood vessels and can cause them to leak fluid, causing blood pressure to drop, blood flow to slow, oxygen and energy to diminish. Infections can be lightning-quick or take their time. They turn a simple leg wound into a three-month stay in Birmingham, with five operations to sort out one rotten artery, and they damage just like shrapnel or bullet – tendons and muscles weakened or ruined, curled toes, months of physio.

Bacteria are everywhere – from the colonies already present on human skin, densest on soldiers from patrol groups who haven't been able to wash much – bacteria that transform in the instant of wounding from domestic nuisance to killer. And then there are the bacteria in the environment in which wars are fought. On the Western Front a millennium of manured farmland ensured that the soil men fell in was rich and dense with every kind of rot bug, and nothing much to fight them with, and in the field hospitals surgeons cut away more and more necrotic flesh, with thoughts of stumps and prosthetics long gone, just trying to save a life, and still the smell of death returned and death itself soon after. Alexander Fleming spent his war in a mobile microbiology lab on the Western Front desperate to solve the problem of the wards that reeked, and the men who rotted away. Afghanistan has its own range of bacteria, either in the desert or in the fertile green zone where the farming is done, and it too got blasted into a casualty on the back of the shrapnel and bomb fragments. Sometimes the soldiers took shelter in a ditch that turned out to be a sewage drain. Blast injury also blew holes in everyone within range, and blew bits of everyone into each other. Someone else's skin bacteria inside them, someone else's bone fragments, their flora-rich intestine, even if whoever is blown up is blown away – gone in a flash – into 'pink mist' – still the bacteria cling to the particle-fines of humanity and look for larger ones to seed.[5] And in a horrifying miniature echo of the Western Front a century before, combatants sometimes smeared excrement and manure on their ammunition and into IEDs so those bacteria buried themselves around bullets and shrapnel in the bodies of their targets.[6] There are lots of fungi in the soil of the green zone, which were particularly problematic for the plastic surgeon, who never forgot about the possibility of fungal infections because they were particularly threatening to the viability of free flaps, and if the Critical Care staff couldn't get them under control with anti-fungals, they reduced the already limited areas that could provide donor tissue.[7]

Not just fungi. Viruses and blood-borne diseases are ever-present in Afghanistan. The malaria season runs from March to the end of October, and soldiers are bad at taking their anti-malarials, so anyone admitted to Bastion and Birmingham during this period was assumed to be at risk, and medication was added to the lines on their body in Critical Care.[8] And then there are those fragments from other bodies that might have been carrying diseases as well as bacteria – hepatitis and HIV in particular. And not just in Afghanistan. In the London bombings of 2007 there were twelve cases where 'biological material implantation' was found to have happened among the casualties, which required complicating testing and treatment at a time when lives hung in the balance.[9] Hospitals too have their own little colonies of bacteria, such as Acinetobacter, hanging around, difficult to totally root out, waiting for intubated Critical Care patients because it likes to roost in their secretions.[10] Use that hand gel the next time you visit a hospital, please, because although there are other reasons why bugs like hospitals, it's the unsanitary practices of visitors that are the worst culprits.

So there are solid, life-saving reasons why the military patients in the Critical Care unit had those endless tests and screens and swabs on anything that leaked out of their body, and their blood and spinal fluid, and tissue samples from debridement surgery, with path labs working flat out, very broad-spectrum antibiotic, anti-fungals all round, and everyone hoping the strains found by the labs weren't resistant. There is a lab in the university next door to the hospital, and there a microbiologist leads teams of researchers trying to push back against the day that all the bugs that can infect a wounded soldier and all the other patients no longer respond to the very broad spectrum they are given on the Critical Care unit. Because that's the day we are back in the foetid tents of the First World War's field hospitals watching the dying, unable to do anything.

Mark Ormrod had a hefty dose of Acinetobacter, and it made him even hotter and more uncomfortable, and it meant that the family who had been able to hold his hand and help him turn over in bed could no longer touch him for fear that they would catch it and spread it around the hospital. So they sat around his bed, hands clasped in their laps, as they were being constantly reminded by the nurses back in their plastic full-length aprons and gloves, and they looked at their son, and he looked back and everyone did a lot of crying, for hours. Once, alone, Mark tried to move himself, for the first time, to roll on to his side without his wounds being scraped as he did so. He had two fingers working on his remaining hand, and so he gripped the bed rail with them and started to pull, and rocked back and forth a little, tensing his weakened stomach muscles to pull himself over, slowly, a little more and a little more, until he could finally lie on his side. He unclawed his fingers from the bed rail and laid his hand carefully down on what was now a rumpled and sweat-sodden bed sheet, the effort utterly exhausting.

Several days later, when he was declared free of the Acinetobacter, his family were allowed to gather close to him, and his father gave him his first shave, so very carefully, from one side of the bed and then across to the other; and as he worked he cried, trying to hide it at first, but then giving in to tears, but keeping his hand with the razor in it always steady. And Mark cried too, and kept his face still until his father was finished, and he told him that soon he'd be shaving himself, he'd see. But every time he closed his eyes for some low-quality sleep, when he woke up all he saw were stumps; no matter how many times he opened his eyes, still stumps. He was not going to wake up and find it was all a bad dream, ever.[11] Mark's own words, own memories. And those of his family too, all of them with the extra second in the chronometry of their lives, the second before waking memory, no going back. They are a strong family, the Ormrods. They seemed instinctively to know what was best for each other. Later, other families would have to be more carefully managed at the bedside. It was too easy to slip into old patterns of parenting, so nurses drew mothers aside and explained that their child was still an adult, even if they were taller than him again, and although they would now have a new life, it would, as far as possible, be an independent one. No matter how hard it was for them to adjust to, they should try. They need not worry about where he was going to sleep from now on or whether they needed to build a wet room. People were going to come and teach their son how to do the things he could not yet quite do on his own, and they should give them some space and let everyone get on with it.

So, gradually, Mark began to look up and see his new road ahead. He knew that his next operation would be his last for that stay (he ate fried chicken and takeaway pizza afterwards to celebrate), and his friends were visiting in numbers. One of them had been a hospital porter and knew his way round all the buildings, and as he chatted, he looked out of Mark's window and realised exactly where they were. He complimented Mark on his inspirational view – of the hospital's morgue. By now Mark could pull himself up enough to look out, and sure enough, just as he did so, an ambulance rolled up and a body was delivered, wrapped in its black plastic shroud.[12] Everyone else in the room laughed, because what else could they do, and Mark watched as the body was wheeled in, until the doors closed behind it and the ambulance pulled away. That was the alternative, a short journey. And now he knew that he preferred the other option, the long journey, the one where he didn't die, with all its pain to be endured, tracking back to life, doors opening, not slamming shut into darkness.

*

But what about when the doors did slam, because the patient had not been able to survive, no matter how hard he was fought for? In the twenty-first century nurses continued to make entries in the patient diary even though they knew their patient would never read it. They told of how they washed him, shaved him, tidied him up. What music had played on the ward radio as they worked, and how they had been honoured to give these last moments of service. The diaries became something entirely for the family left behind. This desire to communicate the care given in a loved one's final hours – to seek somehow to share that process – is nothing new. In 1916, a century before, the first mass conscription armies came to the Western Front, and then followed the first mass conscription deaths in what had become a war of attrition. The medical services were braced for them. Field hospitals with newly dug cemeteries and stacks of plywood coffins, and in between them the moribund wards – what we would today call palliative care (the forerunners of remarkable places like Trinity Hospice)

– where soldiers who could not be saved went to die. Just as at Bastion, they were there for only a few hours, but the nurses, who ran the wards entirely on their own, cared for them every moment, feeling as strongly about them as about any patient they would ever have. They made them comfortable with pain medication or sips of water or just their gentle, skilled company in the last moments. These were never rushed, even if hundreds more men likely to die that day waited for a bed.

Nurses couldn't hold all these moments in their memory, no matter how devoted they were, so they devised a solution (and, unlike at Bastion, we'll never know who by). Special care, went the official directive, should be taken to safeguard the belongings of dying patients. Messages and wishes should be carefully recorded and a special book kept for this purpose.[13] So the belongings were kept in a labelled cotton drawstring bag, and a notebook created – a ward diary – that was taken to each bedside as the patient slipped away or murmured or cried out. For nurses who would have to write as many as sixty 'break the news' letters during offensives to come, the diaries were a godsend. From them they could draw the smallest and most exact details of a life at its end, so that the family had not just a blood-stained uniform and a paybook to remember their loved one by, but a record of their last words, and the scraps of comfort from knowing someone stood at their side to hear them. On the very last day of the war a young soldier died, and his nurse wrote home that

> He passed away peacefully at 5.52 on Tuesday 12th November [...] He talked of going to Blighty to see you and then before he died he thought he was with you all and put out his hands to first one and then the other with such a glad smile, he called you by name and then 'Ada' but we could not catch what else he said. He was a very good patient and we did all we could for him and he had everything that was possible.

Another death, of a much loved regimental medical officer, gave similar details of his end from an abdominal wound, recalled by his nurses weeks after the event for his wife. Without the diary none of this would have been possible.

> Your husband was quite conscious until about 8.30pm and used to ask the conditions of his pulse etc. After about 8.30pm he was unconscious and died at 9.20pm on 20th. He did not speak of anything except, soon after he was admitted, he asked if it would be possible for you to come out, so the MO told him, not so far up the line as this [...] If there is any comfort at all to you, I know your husband did not suffer – in fact he seemed to have no pain at all, only weak and exhausted. I am so very grieved to have to tell you this, because I know just how terrible it all will be to you [...] I am sorry I can tell you so little.

And

> I was with him until almost the last, and, apparently he did not suffer much pain. He was drowsy from the effects of morphia but was quite conscious and took a keen interest in all his symptoms. I think he knew his critical condition but was quite composed and realised that everything possible was being done for him [...] He was anxious to smoke a cigarette which he did about 2 hours before his death. He gradually got weaker from internal haemorrhage and passed peacefully away.[14]

*

The DCCN knew how it was to watch a patient die. In the Critical Care unit at Bastion she had written carefully in their diaries for their families and seen their bodies quietly removed from the ward to the morgue and then home on the aircraft in a flag-draped coffin. She never knew if what she had written had helped, or if it had not helped, or if it had meant nothing. She still doesn't know, and some day she hopes to, but in the meantime she has a note of the days of their death in her own personal diary, one of those with a small leather flap and a lock on it. Every year, on the anniversary, she sits quietly in her office, unlocks the diary, opens the page and remembers each one of them.

15

Mark Ormrod (4)

'How tall are you?'
The Sergeant asked
'Six foot one' I replied
'Bollocks' he retorted …
'You are only as tall
As your rifle …'

'The Great Leveller' by Black Dog[1]

WHEN THE PHYSIO was at Birmingham, he watched Mark Ormrod come in, and worked carefully with the limbs the surgeons had left him with, and watched him be extubated. The physio recalled it for me very clearly, because this was Mark Ormrod, the unexpected survivor: the first, already something of a legend. He'd been among the group of physios who did the assessment of what Mark's rehabilitation would look like, which involved asking Mark what he hoped to get out of the process. Mark had a list ready of the things he wanted to get back to, including running, and the physio remembered thinking what a pity: this patient will have to adjust his expectations of what his life will be from now on.

And then he paused. No, he won't. Those of us who help him with rehabilitation will have to adjust our expectations of what we can deliver, for Mark and for everyone who comes back from the edge and gets all the way to Headley Court. *Choose who you listen to*, Mark would write later, and his physios chose to listen to him.

But Mark had made a tough choice. He'd been six foot one, fifteen stone of lean muscle, never fitter, and now, in his own words, he was a stumpy midget, rifle-tall, who couldn't sit up in bed without help.[2] That was what he learned first: sitting up in bed. Just that. Then, with days of preparation by his physio, getting from his bed into a wheelchair. He had finished his surgeries, but his three stumps were swollen and painful, and he had to try to shift himself on one arm without knocking them. Then sliding down a special board on to the chair. He used muscles to move himself along that he had never used before but that were all that were available to him, and it took an hour. So he and the physio practised over and over until he could do it quicker. One time, on a day when his physio wasn't due, he decided he wanted to get into his chair. The chair was moved in close, and he began the shift. But he over-corrected his balance and started to slip. In the microseconds that passed as he started to fall, he realised that he couldn't land on the floor because the damage to his stumps would mean unbearable pain and probably more surgery, so he grabbed the bars on the bedside and managed somehow to right himself and stay on the bed. Despair, pain and fear – proper fear, not proper in a soldier – but dread of such a small movement, not even a journey really. Waves of pain, sitting, crying but doing it again, until he got into the chair. And then the physio came and they practised some more, and soon Mark was bugging the nurses to let him go outside in the chair.

This meant letting his family see him get into his wheelchair. It also meant going to the flat they were living in while he was in Birmingham and finding that the chair didn't fit through any of the doorways, so the first time he visited he was trapped in the hallway, watching them make dinner for him, so pleased he was there at last, not noticing his anguish and then rushing over when they did. He spent the rest of the evening talking to them through the too-narrow door frames. By the time he next visited he had learned to use his gluteus muscles to extend his hips enough to shuffle along on his bottom, so with tremendous effort he could move around the flat out of his chair, on the floor and through the doorway. He managed to shuffle across the living-room carpet over to where the sofa was and sat leaning up against it on the floor, working out how to get up on to it. He was determined to get up there without help and to sleep there that night, and not back at the hospital. He got up on to it, but the effort it took to travel six feet across the room and lift his body weight up on to a sofa using his one good arm drained him completely. He remembers this being his lowest point since he begged a friend to finish him off in the bloody dust of Afghanistan.

Then his girlfriend sat down beside him and spoke of his achievements so far, how the physios were astounded at his progress, how they would have a life together, guiding Mark back up to a place from which he could move forward again. And then, a few days later, the prosthetics expert from Headley Court came to assess Mark's stumps, followed quickly by a double amputee who briefed him on what it was like to have a state-of-the-art prosthetic fitted entirely for him, with micro-processors to control the hydraulics, and told him that the chances were he could live without a wheelchair in his life at all, just the legs. And Mark chose to believe him as he watched him walk out of his room on just the legs, walking well and firmly. Mark's future: walking like that out of the room, six foot one again, walking out of all the rooms he wanted to, with no more sobbing on the floor or doorways he couldn't get through.

16

Rehabilitation: Headley Court

IN A MEDICAL CONTEXT, rehabilitation means restoring a human being to effectiveness by training after injury, disease or surgery. Rehabilitation is a specialised form of healthcare, focusing on the achievement of the highest levels of function and independence and quality of life. For the patients of the military ward at Birmingham, the unexpected survivors of the Afghan cohort, including Mark Ormrod, this specialised form of healthcare was done at Headley Court. Headley Court, in Surrey, has been the centre of military rehabilitation services since the Second World War. But the roots of rehabilitation, wherever it is done in Britain today, lie in the First World War, with all those orthopaedic specialists who took their understanding of locomotor systems out to the casualties of the Western Front and restored their lives. How we understand physical rehabilitation today comes from them, word for word, across a century.

In the last months of the First World War, Sir Robert Jones reflected on the work that he and his orthopaedic colleagues had done, and what it meant for medicine as a whole. He emphasised how what they did was never just about repair. They all had 'an orthopaedic mind which thinks in terms of function, and has to deal with a pre-operative and post-operative stage as well as an operative stage, which although it may be essential, has only a proportional value'.[1] Surgery was just one part of the process. Surgery alone would not be sufficient to restore a human being to effectiveness. Of equal importance was 'the treatment by manipulation, operation and re-education of disabilities of the locomotor system'.[2]

Jones had built his network of orthopaedic centres on these principles, creating rehabilitation centres 'with operative, technical and re-educational departments'.[3] Inside these departments specialist therapists trained their patients in movements that made everything in the system stronger: not just bones but muscles and nerves and joints too. The careful rebuilding of muscle power within a smashed and reconstructed locomotor system, using exercises, repetitive stretches, massages. Jones included a range of different skills within these departments: physiotherapists, massage therapists, the electro-therapists, the hydrotherapists, gymnasium therapists (therapists who designed rehabilitation around gymnastic equipment such as ropes and wall bars and got kit specially made if it didn't do exactly what they needed it to).[4] Everyone working together to create a new locomotor system, with the wreckage of the old one. For the majority of the patients who passed through his centres the ultimate aim was to support the fitting of the often delicate and complicated artificial limbs produced in the prosthetics workshop by instrument makers (we don't call them that today, and I rather wish we did), to restore the wearer 'to the highest possible grade of health and earning power'. Or function and independence – however you like to put it. As I like to put it, one hundred years later, welcome to Headley Court.

*

Rehabilitation: it's not surgery, it's exercises. Everything's slower. There's none of the urgency of the cabin of a helicopter swerving through hostile fire, rushing back to Bastion, or the brilliance amid the chaos of the trauma bays. By the time rehab began, everyone's lives were saved, blood back where it should be, point zero way off in the distance. Negotiations over, the deal was done. There was no blood on the floor or life measured in pulse beats on a monitor. The patient didn't die. Nobody dies at Headley Court. But rehab doesn't mean that the hard part is over. It's all the same hard part, from point of wounding to rehabilitation. What happens at Headley is a continuation of what was started in the desert, with a tourniquet or a field dressing or a chest drain. No point in having one without the other.

Like Bastion, everything was transformed at Headley after 2009. Before then, Headley ran along quietly, managing military rehabilitation that mostly meant sports injuries – soldiers running, playing rugby, climbing – pushing themselves too far and wanting to get back to doing it in double-quick time. There was capacity to spare, so it also treated locals, referred by the NHS (Robert Lawrence did his head injury rehab at Headley and met a girlfriend there with a sports injury). But once the IEDs began to infest the landscape of Afghanistan there were no more spare beds for civilians or the lightly injured as, for the first time in almost fifty years, Headley found itself overmatched. Injuries, particularly blast injuries, required an immediate response. So all the physios they could fit in were hired, from inside and outside the military. A new residential unit was built because there wasn't enough room in the old house, and the existing buildings grew: the gym, the prosthetics workshop, the car park, scattered about the grounds, wherever space, time and the planning system allowed.

And although we aren't really allowed to say this sort of thing as historians, it was as if everything at Headley had been waiting, gathering together exactly what was needed just in time. All those sports physios and rehab specialists, all their work oriented to getting young, determined soldiers back running, playing rugby, skiing. They had little experience of anything else, so that's what they brought into the treatment rooms and the gym every day. Get back to where their patients were before they were injured, somehow, despite what has been lost. This is not how it works outside the military. NHS rehab tends to focus on what has been left, rather than what can be regained, which isn't wrong necessarily; it's just the way it is. Things have evolved differently in a system that has to treat everything from car crashes to diabetic complications to bad backs. By 2010 the difference was officially enshrined at Headley, where 'the outcome goals for service personnel after injury are considerably higher than those set within civilian practice.'[5]

Headley is not a hospital. At Headley the patients are dressed, and they've been home, and so to them it feels like the next stage, where everything will be different. Perhaps they aren't even patients any more, not entirely, even if they still have IVs for antibiotic drips and analgesia some of the time. The good part of its being different is that Headley is the place where they start to take on responsibility for their recovery, in partnership with physios and prosthetists. There's a hard part of being different as well. Coming to Headley makes them realise that, despite the weeks and months at Birmingham, there are problems that are not yet fixed, and that fixing them completely may not be one of the available options.

Headley is where all the difficult, serious, hard questions are asked for the first time. What is happening to me? What is going to happen to me? Where do I fit in from now on? Who am I now? And Headley is where the pain really rolls in when they thought it was gone, and the phantoms catch up with them, and their brain doesn't normalise and the last bits of their old sense of self slip away. There are mirrors everywhere at Headley. Huge walls full of them, in which people with new lives to comprehend stare at their reflection, at the price of the deal; there is no getting away from it.

Coming to Headley could feel strange right from the start. The entrance is via a courtyard surrounded by the walls and high, darkened windows of the Jacobean house, and some people find it spooky, which is fair enough because in one of the windows there hangs a skeleton, slowly twisting on a hook.

The window belongs to the office of one of the rehab specialists, who needs the skeleton because obviously it's the best way to demonstrate the interconnectivity of bones, but when people walked or wheeled into this whole new world, strange trumped obvious every time. Their family came with them into their new room, and put their stuff in drawers or in wardrobes, sponge bags in the small bathroom with the disabled fittings, and went to whatever meetings they were allowed to, but soon they went home, leaving them behind.

Then came their first real meeting with them at its centre. They sat in a group, one part of what was introduced as a multi-disciplinary team – nurses, pain consultants, rehab consultants, physios, prosthetists (sounded good), a mental health specialist (couldn't see why they were there). The meeting resulted in two things. A problem list. And then, based on that, and quickly, because otherwise the mental health specialist knew where that went, a series of goals. The only ones they really remembered to tell the historian about were the ones they set for themselves, and it was usually roughly the same one for all, no matter how long the problem list – I want to run again. Scott Meenagh had two: he wanted to be on his big legs by July, and running by Halloween. Personal goals, big goals, and so they were noted, at the top of the page on their file, but so were other smaller goals (like 'do stairs') because in the weeks to come they would need to see small targets met on the way to bigger ones. As it says in the textbook: patients may need encouragement and support to improve their performance, but the more difficult cases to manage require a limitation to be placed on their activity – a common phenomenon in high-achieving military or sporting personnel. Sometimes doing too much is as dangerous as doing too little: both do damage. Acceptance, understanding, 'concordance' – a medical term which means agreement, but which sounds bigger than that because in this context it is.[6]

They'd seen themselves in mirrors before – they had them in bathrooms at Birmingham and when they got home – but the mirrors at Headley are huge, covering whole walls, and the lighting is bright and hard and real. The mirrors at home were something they looked in alone, at pieces of themselves, trying to put things together. Their first sight of themselves full length – not full-length – was hard, but at Headley there was someone else there with them, usually a physio, also looking, pointing out something interesting on their new selves – postural re-education, gait re-education – and before long they could see it themselves, could keep tabs on how they were doing, precisely, competitively, like they did before. Mirrors – they think about them on burns wards because that first sight of the new self has to be carefully managed, so nothing in the bathrooms, nothing reflective or shiny at all, but patients still try to see themselves in the back of spoons, in reflections on metal teapots, on glass door panels. Not at Headley. There was their new self, right there, all along the walls of the gym and the treatment rooms, every step they took reflected back at them. Using this method to accept a new self wasn't an initiative from the mental health end of their team. It was, as any physio will tell you (and one told me), very important to adjust, to see the wound and see what was left of them. Since the age of two, their brain and body had worked in sync – sensory feedback and a learned movement pattern. Twenty-something years later, and deployment to Afghanistan, and it was all gone, and so they needed to learn a new one, and to learn, they needed to see.[7] It got so they looked forward to seeing it, because at the same time they could see their own progress, right there in the mirror.

Not everything was unfamiliar and had to be relearned from the brain up. This was medical treatment, but it was also a new posting. Back in the military, back at work, back on duty, tasked with something. Almost everyone at Headley is in military uniform, and there was saluting, and hats to be worn at the right time and in the right place. They showed their ID cards when entering and leaving the grounds to duty sergeants in guardhouses. This wasn't the annoying RAF nit-picking; this was proper medical reckoning. Their recovery was now their military service, so they should act like it. They were becoming a soldier again, even though in the long weeks at Birmingham it never really felt like they would be. At Headley they were a soldier again, so they should try to look like one, cut their hair really short again, clean regimental T-shirt, try to feel like one. Back in the army, with regulations they recognised and had come to rely on, and were relying on again. Even if they couldn't quite find their new self yet, there was structure left over from the old one to fall back on in the meantime.

17

Sockets and Stumps

A HEADLEY PATIENT'S FIRST STAY usually lasted twenty-four days. When the physios and everyone in the team agreed, people from the prosthetics department arrived, and that was always a very good day. Prosthetics are the artificial substitutes for parts of the human body that are missing. Prosthetics can be permanently implanted (teeth, facial bones, hips, knee joints) or removable (hand, arm, leg). Like the rest of this book, this chapter focuses mostly on removable prosthetic legs, because it is prosthetic legs that represent the greatest challenge to both builder and wearer. Legs need to be load-bearing, to carry their wearer forward, to get them up and out of the chair for as long as possible. Other prosthetics do other things for their wearer, but none has quite the same impact, or quite the same level of technical difficulty, as getting them up and out of their wheelchair.

Prosthetics in one form or another have been around as long as human beings have had the wit to build them. For most of lost-limb history, they've been made of wood, carved to shape and lumped around, strapped around whatever is left of the body part they were meant to replace. The modern prosthetic leg, jointed and with metal and wood parts as we would recognise it today, evolved for the two largest amputee cohorts produced in war: 38,000 from the American Civil War and (in Britain) 41,000 from the First World War. War didn't just produce amputees and legs for its casualties; it also produced prosthetic limb industries – workshops, research, design studios, manufacturing and fitting. And durable, limbs as well as organisations. Many of the companies that were successful in the nineteenth and twentieth centuries are still market leaders today in the twenty-first (more about one in particular later). Today most people know about the extraordinary gains in prosthetic technology from events such as the Paralympics, where materials and design technologies are brought together to produce performance limbs for superhumans.[1]

Prosthetic limbs, and in particular prosthetic legs, have come to represent everything we know about dealing with amputation. This isn't quite right, because the limb that we can see is only the end, not the means whereby amputees are able to function. Also, because despite all the research and development and superhuman efforts, prosthetic limbs don't work as well as we would like. A design historian summed this up elegantly (as design historians are wont to do): 'of all machines [the artificial limb] has the closest proximity with the human body but the least chance of matching its performance.'[2] The primary reason for the generally sub-optimal performance of artificial limbs is not the artificial limb itself but the stump on to which it fits. It fits on to the stump by means of a socket, and it is this system that is at the heart of limb replacement. Which is why this chapter is called 'Sockets and Stumps' rather than 'Prosthetic Legs'.

Meanwhile, back to the team meeting at Headley where the amputee first met the prosthetics department (a private company, Blatchfords, by the way, founded in 1890 and greatly expanded during the First World War, responsible for a model of leg prosthetic named 'The Clapper', because that was the sound it made when fully extended; at least the models are silent now). In the twenty-first century the prosthetist took the bandages off their patient's stumps and looked really closely at them, handling the stumps in a different way from everyone before, as something to work with, with potential. If there was no infection, and they were healing normally, and the work in the gym was going to plan, then they came back with a load of kit, including a bucket full of plaster cast. Then they covered the stumps in cling film and took a plaster cast mould.

In the prosthetists' workshop, where they do more of these for highly demanding, impatient humans than anywhere else in the country, they think that plaster cast moulds are still more efficient than a digital scan and 3D printed models. So far, even the best computer scanner isn't a match for a really experienced prosthetist with an artist's eye and a set of fine files to reshape carefully until the fit is as good as it can be. The kit associated with making plaster casts can make the prosthetic workshop look like a sculptor's studio. There are five prosthetists at Headley, and they all have white plaster residue in their fingernail beds and knuckles, and they all make very slightly different-looking casts, so anyone who knows how they work can tell who built which model, like telling a Michelangelo from a Bernini.[3]

In the workshop they make a hard-plug solid replica of the stump. And from the solid replica they make a bucket-shaped object that slots over the stump: a socket. And everything that has gone in this book before comes down to this piece of machinery, a socket, carefully honed to fit a human, and to the moment when it is first handed over (and it's heavier than it looks – as heavy as the original body part it is to replace because that's what the central nervous system is used to). They are not handing over a leg. They are handing over the means to a leg. The dictionary says a socket is a natural or artificial hollow for something to fit into or stand firm, or that can be used to make a connection.

So this is the beginning of a long journey together, not just a handover and a fitting, and most of the journeys begun in 2009 are still going on. Their patients will learn to call them 'my prosthetist', and no one will ever look at them as carefully as they do, except the patients themselves. They say things like, 'Oh you've got a lovely residual limb', which means the plastic surgeon and the physios and the negative pressure dressings and the wraps have all delivered them a stump they can work with. It isn't weird, it's good, so the patients adjust to the prosthetist's mindset and then communication begins. Good communication, thinking about every word that is said to them to explain how they are feeling, what they see in the mirror. They learn precision communication about precision movement, and they learn not to hold back anything, because it saves time and pain.[4] The only thing prosthetists never want to see in their workshop is soldiers suffering in silence, keeping quiet and bleeding into their sockets. Not helpful, ever, in or out of the workshop.

Sockets aren't just about something to clip a limb into. They restore evenness of length to limbs, because blast injury rarely gives them anything neat to work with. Stumps are of different volumes, different widths and different lengths. Sockets have inner linings that even things up and make things steady.[5] An amputated thigh bone (femur) floats about in the soft tissue of the thigh itself, without muscles and ligaments to hold it effectively where it should be. So the socket has to fit closely over the stump and give shape, structure in such a way that the whole thing is made stable, with no more floating about, doing damage. The socket needs to be not too tight and not too loose: just right to hold the stump in a new place, firmly, all the time.

Part of this stability is about the weight of the rest of the body and how that comes down on to the stump. Bone that has been cut through can't take weight, so the socket is designed to take the weight of the body and distribute it back to areas with soft and hard tissue intact. Generally, this means the weight is moved through the socket structure to areas that can carry it, such as the hips and pelvis. So each stump, even on the same patient, is different because no two stumps are ever the same, not after 2009. Depending on the bone, and how the blast has blown it away, the socket may go high up the leg, almost to the hip to provide the support to the soft tissue and leftover muscles. It's really complicated stuff, and never exactly, pre-cisely, permanently right.

So 80 per cent of the prosthetist's time with the patient will be about getting the sockets as right as humanly pos-sible. Sometimes what's right in the morning is wrong by the evening, leaving a blister or a patch rubbed red and raw, or swelling in the repairs made so carefully by the plastic surgeon. When the socket is first fitted, it's left on for a while and then taken off again. They stare down at it, and wait for any red marks left behind to fade away. If after ten minutes the marks are still visible, then the socket needs work, so back they go to the cast, and the set of tools, and they work looking back and forth from the stump to the socket, and then they try again. Most people got a new socket or major socket work done at least once a month after their original fitting. It's like a new pair of shoes that pinch at the end of the first day you wear them, even though you really want to wear them because they are new. And the next day, blisters, so you have to wear an old pair or trainers because of the pain.

But with sockets, not being able to put them on because of a graze or a blister or swelling meant going back in the chair. Stumps changed after they'd come back from their week off away from the gym, gone home, got hungry, started eating again and so been fed from morning until night by families grateful to see their progress. Out with friends, pubs, beer. Even slight fluctuations in weight affected the volume of the stump, and suddenly, really annoyingly, the socket no longer fitted. Some people have different stump volumes every morning and every evening, no matter what they do or don't do. Humans swell and shrink as they get hot or cold, and fluid shifts around their body, particularly a body that has been assaulted and bat-tered at the molecular level by blast injury. Just the simple act of sweating – the means whereby a body regulates its own tem-perature – is problematic with stump and socket. The socket traps the sweat, heat builds up, sweat accumulates, dirt accu-mulates in the sweat, and then the carefully repaired tissue on the stump softens – 'macerates', to give it its technical name – and then damage is done.[6]

But, for all of that, it was a great moment when the pair of elasticated socks that act as a liner between stump and socket was handed over for the first time. The patient padded out the gaps in their own scarred flesh to make it even, and then rolled them over their stump, handling it like the expert that everyone at Headley had helped them become. Sprayed the socks with some liquid that made them fit, and then on with the socket. Fitted like a dream, stayed on with a vacuum seal. It felt tight, always, the first time, as the flesh was enclosed and pressure started to take the strain and move the weight around. Then they looked down, and they no longer saw battered, bulbous remnants but two neat stumps, dressed and ready for business. And beside them the prosthetist smiled – just a small one, because although so much more work would be needed, this was still special.

Next stop: standing. Sockets can't be stood on, and something needs to be clipped on to their ends that is suitable for standing. But going straight to a long prosthetic is very demanding, not only in terms of balance and mobility but also in terms of the immense effort required metabolically. So the solution is to go gradually, starting with a foreshortened prosthetic – 'stubbies', as they are more commonly known. A stub at the end of a stump, not yet a length. Stubbies have a clip that goes on to the socket and then a couple of inches of connection length with a rounded flat disk on the bottom. When patients stand, stubbies are what they first stand on, and it feels like not much effort at all, because their centre of gravity is low, so balance and stability are easy, and although their steps are short, the effort required to make them is not too much – heart rate stays low, less sweating into the socket, all round a good thing. Stairs are difficult in stubbies, but generally they are the prosthetic version of bedroom slippers. Something comfortable that can be relied on, although not always, according to one of their manufacturers, 'cosmetically appealing' (stubbies, not slippers). Stubbies won't make them as tall as their rifle again, but they are a significant move forward.

Scott Meenagh was up on his stumps and stubbies three days after arriving at Headley. Mark Ormrod was asked to stand still while the prosthetic people marked up his socket for some minor adjustments. No chance, he was never standing still again unless it was on a parade ground or at his wedding, so the prosthetists could work while he was moving his weight from thigh to thigh, almost walking.[7] Getting better was exciting, the first real positive personal excitement they'd had for a while.[8] But the team had to be very careful at this stage, because their patients could easily start to overdo it, really pushing themselves in the gym, as their stubbies allowed them to use weights, stand up, develop the core and abs and joints, everything that hadn't been blown up or removed by a surgeon.

Stubbies make the next stage much easier. The next stop will be big legs, as they call them at Headley (soldiers rename everything: crutches are comfy sticks). Big legs are the same length and weight as the leg that has gone, so they are tall again, taller than their mum. They haven't rushed on to big legs because there's one important thing to remember about big legs (or any prosthetic limb), and that is: the longer it is, the more complicated, the more difficult to master and the more expensive. Below the knee (a flesh wound, as they like to call it at Headley), prosthetics are pretty straightforward. Through the knee is more difficult, but what's left of the joint can be incorporated into a socket design and every little helps with the new movement range. Above the knee is hardest of all. Nothing to work with, movement forward will come from the rest of the body, hips and pelvis, very hard.

And pretty soon into 2009 the staff at Headley understood this better than anyone, so word went out all the way back to the surgeons at Bastion. Give us as much bone to work with as possible, amputate low and keep everything long. Whatever can be spared, physios and prosthetists can work with. And the surgeons took note and changed their practice – as much bone as they could save sent home, below the knee where possible, through the knee likewise (although it's a much more complicated surgical technique), above the knee only where life hung in the balance. Robert Jones had, of course, said it all before:

> One point which has impressed all who are seeing end results is the necessity that we should work in much closer association with surgeons [at the Front]. In this way we could approach problems from their point of view, and they would learn also of the later phases of their cases. It would strengthen judgement on both sides, and clarify and standardize treatment. Consultants on both sides of the Channel would find it a welcome relief to share each other's burdens.[9]

Surgeons and physios who worked at Bastion and Headley are still sharing that lesson and so, hopefully, the burdens of their colleagues today. In July 2016 the first of what will be a regular course teaching the techniques of through-knee amputations was held by orthopaedic surgeons from Bastion for surgeons from Cambodia, the Philippines, Indonesia, Ethiopia, Kenya, Mexico, Lebanon and Sri Lanka who are dealing with the aftermath of legacy minefields, in numbers that greatly exceed that of the Afghan cohort.[10]

No matter where in the world, especially Headley, with all the mirrors, the first few steps taken on 'big legs' weren't particularly dignified. The big leg prosthetic itself was locked on to the socket fixture, but initially to keep it on there was a kind of harness in neoprene and Velcro, wrapped around the patient by the physio. Getting up on to the socket with the legs on was too hard for them to do on their own at first. In the early days the solution was a kind of mini-crane, with the patient clipped on then hoisted up and into position between a set of parallel bars; this held them there while they grabbed on and let the weight slowly come down through the sockets on to the legs. By 2010 the crane was wheeled out of the gym and the physios lifted their patients up themselves, one between two, and gently down on to the sockets. And whichever way it happened, usually when they looked up from between the bars, their families were there crying and taking all the photos their phones could handle because they were tall again, and it suddenly didn't matter about all the webbing and the straps and the crane. This was it.[11]

And then cracking on (as every soldier I have ever met always says). The terrain between those two parallel bars became everything in their life. They could probably map it: the dents in the reinforced plastic handles, every single ripple in the mat on the floor, the sounds as their feet dragged when they shouldn't, their breathing, heavy and hard, effortful, but slowly getting more even. Back and forth, back and forth, turn round and back again. Strain, strength, sweat in their socket, maceration, pain, parallel bars, new life. In all the photographs of them they are wearing their pushing gloves – the ones they were first given at Birmingham, which they put on when they had to start learning how to use a wheelchair. Now they use them to protect their hands on the parallel bars – much better – they don't mind having them on in the photographs at all.

Big legs were starter legs. Fairly basic, just for learning to get up and stay up and move. Everyone knew what came next, and it was the high point of a journey where previously they thought there had no high points. The next steps would be taken on those really expensive legs that were tailor-made in the prosthetics workshop for them from socket fix to foot section. It really is a workshop, nothing remotely medical about it – and if earlier I compared it to a sculptor's studio, it might also be a garage for a Formula One vehicle, which, in a way, it is. The lightest materials, brilliant technicians and the kind of design that means patients can have their limbs any way they want, in the future, even knock up a couple of shin pads on a 3D printer at home to match their jacket and shorts (not quite there yet, but it's not as far away as you might think).

The really expensive stuff is in the knee joint. There are sensors all over the legs measuring what's going on, and they send signals to a microprocessor tucked into the knee bend, and the microprocessor directs hydraulics to control the knee joint. The microprocessor is going to replace the twenty-odd years of sensory feedback from body to brain and make something new that works for limbs that weren't always there. The whole central nervous system has to get used to a unit on the back of the new leg. It won't be easy, but the effect is transformative: without knees, things like stairs become mountains. To lift up each leg, with a prosthetic attached, to go up a stair and then another and another, the amputee can only call on muscle groups at their hips and lower back. The actual lift arc that can be achieved is no more than inches, so going upstairs means swinging the whole leg around and over the top of each stair, and then hauling the rest of the body up too.

There's a technical term for it: hip-walking. It is doubly difficult for the double amputee, swinging back and forth, stump drifting in the socket, a high arc of movement. Friction, heat and pain. The normal, confident, paced walk along a straight line with no one really noticing they are on prosthetics is broken for the shift to going upstairs. Everyone has to slow down, gather up the muscles they need around their body; everyone tries not to look or be looked at; everyone has to remember always, every day. They have to ask questions whether there will be stairs, and how many of them, and then have the difficult, unwelcome conversation about lifts. So a knee with a microprocessor can be transforming. Sensory data is gathered up from all over their leg, the new one and the old one. Things like gait and speed and surface. It learns to recognise the impulses that say what muscles are used for movement and what it means when they activate them. It's not ideal: microprocessors need to deliver control strategies for how the legs manage at speed, on a variety of surfaces and for the kind of complicated gaits that the amputation has left them with. This little computer, which is replacing so much of their central nervous system, needs to recognise when they've stopped. It needs to be able to put their legs in the kind of holding patterns ('conscious standing function') that are needed for standing still or sitting down, or leaning. Something that allows them to get going again without too much effort to hitch up and off. And preferably do it in a way that doesn't drain the batteries, because these kinds of legs need charging, so every time battery technology gets better, so do legs. And going upstairs is one thing. How about being able to walk backwards? And manage all the transitions – sit to stand to walk, walk to run, step over step upstairs and down, with no other compensating movements. So the new long leg was complicated, and wouldn't deliver everything its owners wanted, but for all that they felt better the first time they saw them at Headley. And sometimes the prosthetic people liked a bit of drama, so they didn't always tell them theirs were ready – they just made a normal appointment for some socket-tweaking, and they walked in and there were the legs, in the middle of the workshop, spray laminate coating glittering in a spotlight, and the patients' spirits soared.

Then they put them on for the first time, and it suddenly wasn't quite so straightforward. The really expensive legs were difficult to get used to – the sensors and microprocessors learning their new owner as much as their new owner was learning them. It felt like a step back, not confident steps forward. It felt like many steps back or, worse, no steps at all. Like learning to ride a bicycle. We can all remember that. The moment your training wheels are off and the hands of your family are pulled back (most of the way hovering near your back, but you can't see that because they are behind you), and you have to go forward on your own, on the thin wheels with only your own brain doing the complicated balancing thing. That long second when you can't quite bring yourself to push forward, when your memory reminds you of grazes and bleeding and plasters, but there's too much at stake and so somehow your brain makes contact with the right muscles and the pedals turn and you move and you don't fall. You don't go very far, but it's far enough, and you never forget how to do that again. And behind you, your family cry a little bit and take a billion photographs. It's exactly like that, except it's a first step, and there are no pedals: just the patient and the new version of their central nervous system, acting in tandem.

The first time on long legs, walking, reminded them that they had really forgotten how to do something that they thought they had mastered as toddlers. Falling. And the more and the further they moved, the more likely they were to fall. The prosthetics manufacturers know this (which is why some of their R&D comes under the heading 'optimised stumble recovery'). So learning to walk became learning not to be afraid of falling, not minding and getting up again. Physios teach humans who no longer have all their original joints to care for those that are left. Before, when they fell, they put their hands out, palms down, to break their fall. But now they may not have both hands. And even if they do have both, falling damages wrists, elbows and shoulders, none of which they can afford to have out of action as they learn their prosthetics. So they learned to fall like a stuntman, starting on crash mats piled up in the gym, automatically going into a roll, dispersing the impact of hitting the ground on to their trunk, the least worst place for it to go on their new body.

Although Headley is recognised as world-class in the NHS and beyond, on one metric they failed constantly. Falling. People aren't supposed to fall in hospital, because mostly they are over sixty-five and falling makes everything worse. Only at Headley did every fall teach the patients something, get them up faster; there are limits to NHS statistics, so move on and don't worry about it.

18

Mark Ormrod (5)

MARK ORMROD was in the prosthetics workshop on his second day at Headley, getting cast up for his sockets. He'd been told at Birmingham that he would be working his arse off at rehab to walk again, but he hadn't done that exactly because, as physios had explained, what arse muscles he had left were vital to recovery. Of the many things he found out about himself in his first twenty-four days at Headley, he was finding the chair was not a place he wanted to be, ever. He was also trying to be a parent again, but in the chair and with only one arm, this was becoming the hardest and most frustrating part.[1]

He had a daughter, born before his injury, whom he saw on the one week in four away from Headley. By the end of it he felt like an utter failure as a father and sometimes a danger, because he couldn't care for her the way he wanted to. She was small and already walking well, but she still fell down occasionally and hurt herself. Every time he had to ask someone to get to her, to pick her up and to bring her over and put her in his lap, and he had to have parked the chair in the meantime somewhere stable enough for him to use his one arm to comfort her, to tell her it would be all right, and then somehow work out how to help her back down to the ground, where she could run off again. Every time he felt anger if whoever could pick her up and bring her over didn't do it immediately, when every second she cried in someone else's arms felt so much longer. Anger because every time he came back and saw her she could run further away from him and do more, like swimming or hide-and-seek, and he could do none of it. He couldn't even spend time with her, just the two of them. And he could see into the future: a future where, once she was big enough, she would end up pushing him around.

He took that anger back to rehab and channelled it into getting out of the chair and re-learning all the things that his daughter could do better than him, so he could be a dad again. He was quick, really quick considering he was the first triple they had had at Headley, which was its own challenge. So he did what he was told, to the max, Marine-style and was up on his stumps six weeks after the explosion.[2] Rattling through each stage. Big legs, cranes and Velcro, family taking pictures. Smiles and stubbies, up and down, walking, working. Then the long legs moment in the spotlight of the workshop. Fitting, gym, positioned back between the parallel bars, battery on the microprocessor fully charged and sensors engaged. Then a deep breath moment, a long extra second, everything about to change. All that speed, to this point.

And he found that this point was sharp, and scary, suddenly suspended above the prosthetic, as if he would smash down on his stumps at any moment. And he was frightened, really frightened, more than he had ever been in his life – and that included anything Afghanistan had found to throw at him. He couldn't bring himself to move, and he was the only one who could change that. No medics, no helicopter in the distance coming to lift him away, no physios, no one else. If he fell now, everything would get so much worse, and really, how could anything have been worse? Back down, to the place that he loathed more than anywhere else, the place where he had no power, and he couldn't stay there, so he didn't. Choose who you listen to. Choose not to listen to the fear. Choose a different part of his brain. Activate it, move muscles, weight, and then the sensors picked it up and the knee joint worked and the leg bent as it should and he moved forward. Struggle, balance, don't fall, didn't fall, struggle, balance again.

And so Ormrod worked, and bent his knees, and shouted at them to work, and walked and stood, taller than his rifle again, because he was getting married to the girl who had sat beside him on the floor and brought him back from desolation, and he was going to be a dad who could pick up his children and a husband who had walked up the aisle at their wedding and, later on, who danced with his wife, to their song ('Amazed', by Lonestar, in case you are wondering).

19

A Short History of Headley Court and Its Garden

(neither of which is as old as it looks)

WHEN THE FIRST TWENTY-FOUR DAYS have passed, the patients at Headley have time to look around them and wonder at its strangeness. Headley looks like a perfect Jacobean master-piece, conceived by a gentleman creative genius some time in the 1700s. Except it wasn't. It was originally a pretty ordinary farmhouse, bought and rebuilt by a very newly rich Victorian, Walter Cunliffe, at the end of the nineteenth century, and he didn't much care for Gothic or Arts and Crafts or any of the prevailing aesthetics, so instead he made a grand house from a period he did like, built by the architect Edward Warren, copying the styles of two hundred years before, including a huge and weirdly wonderful garden. There are even features that imply actual Jacobean presences – the Pepys door to the billiard room – and the Cromwell Room, which has panelling on the walls that came originally from a house owned by the Lord Protector's sister.

The panelling bought Cromwell's ghost with it, apparently.

The Lord Protector floats about through the walls, and even today medics and patients talk about feeling his presence as they work late or walk dark corridors alone. Perhaps he means to be there, observing what he started. It was on his watch, during the English Civil War, that a bill was passed recognising the government's duty of care to the soldiers killed or wounded in its service.[1] The first dedicated military hospital opened in London as a result, and then two more, staffed by doctors and nurses recruited from among the widows of soldiers. A short experiment but a precedent set. Restoration in 1660 meant repudiation and closure for any institutions created in the Interregnum, with responsibility for military healthcare reverting to individual regimental colonels, although the building of the Royal Hospital at Chelsea went some way to redressing the old wounds.

Inside even the new buildings, more strangeness. Part of one of the gyms at Headley, its walls covered in mirrors, had a wide yellow track painted on the floor that wound through the whole area. It wasn't a metaphor, it had a practical purpose: so that everyone knew not to leave things lying on the track, because that was where people walked on their big legs for the first time, and they needed the way to be clear. But the metaphor is irresistible. Follow the yellow brick road, where the wizard at the end turns out to be their own reflection. And it was good the first couple of times, but then what the patients mainly found was that the yellow brick road, and the gym, were no longer enough. They were too small, too busy and not real. Real life has things left in the way, and where they can't decide entirely where they slow down or speed up. Real decides where and when, and real is better. Then they looked out of the windows and noticed that the garden was real, all around, so they stepped through the doors of the main house, and went to find it.

In 1912 *Country Life* magazine came to Headley to write a feature about the house. It was probably the crowning moment of its architect's life, although, like so much else in the period, what the article did was capture part of the British way of life that would soon be blasted away in the First World War. They wrote about everything, including the bits of Cromwelliana, but they particularly liked the garden. So do I, and because it looks today much like it did then, here's what they said (and it's hard to resist a bit of Edwardian lifestyle magazine language):

> Headley Court is approached from the north along a broad drive flanked by well-trimmed yew hedges. The south side [...] is laid out as a large lawn, broken by topiary work. The main gardens lie on the north-east side and are made the more interesting by the provision of a great bathing pond. A practical point with regard to the pergola pillars is also worth noting. They are of grey slate, which has weathered to the colour of sea-worn oak and has the great advantage that it is, for all practical purposes, everlasting. Very attractive, too, are the many lead figures which have been employed. There is one gay-looking person busy with pipe and drum. In a fountain basin in the north-east garden several chubby little boys sit on over-turned vases [...] and at the south-west two classical figures keep watch over the big yew sundial. In the lower walled garden there is another sundial of very original design. Among the most striking features of the gardens are the yew hedges; those surrounding the lawn are broken at regular intervals by wedge-shaped clumps or buttresses of clipped golden yew projecting into the lawn and giving an admirable contrast of colour.

They weren't exaggerating about the big yew sundial. It takes up a whole lawn, all the numbers, precisely located, even the gnomon – the part that casts the shadow – and the family who commissioned it probably never even saw it fully grown. But everyone at Headley in its twenty-first-century life knows it well. Gigantic sundial, taller than a man on his long legs, and it only tells someone the time if they go up a ladder or look out of one of the upstairs windows. The yew hedges and walls make long corridors, to private places, past topiary rabbits and trains. There's an orchard, cherries and apples, for the big house, and a nuttery (but no one has called it that for at least fifty years because it's never a helpful word in a place with a designated psychiatric unit), with hazel and cobnut trees. And a proper Victorian greenhouse, for delicate plants and vegetables, just like in *Downton Abbey*. Nothing is hard or too formal, just carefully shaped to lead the visitor around the place, pleasingly. It was a wonderful mind that made that garden. Even the bricks in the walls are beautiful, and the walls themselves contain and define the garden, not in a confining, wall-y way, just evenly paced breaths, as those who come here look out, letting their brain make sense of it one component at a time. Walls, beautifully made and placed, walls can set people free, at their own pace, and calmly, no worrying about what lies beyond the horizon.

In 1987 the hurricane that struck the south of England took away many of the really big trees, and they were replaced by flat, cheaply maintained lawn, but the yew hedges were untouched and the garden didn't really change its overall form. The remaining panes of glass in the greenhouse were smashed, and weeds grew up and out of it, and the topiary got a bit straggly, especially the rabbits, and the orchard trees went unpruned.[2] But it was still essentially the same place that *Country Life* had photographed in 1912. Somehow, despite the destruction, still a place full of unusual and fanciful elements, according to the post-storm survey, with 'the remnants of an exceedingly interesting garden'.[3] Remnants are something they know their way around at Headley.

Like everyone else at Headley in 2009, the garden made itself useful immediately. It turns out there was a whole harvest of new goals growing amid the walls if patients and therapists knew where to look for them. There is a long grassy slope down to the main lawn. Getting up and down it on new long legs became the main metric to successful prosthetic fitting and use. No acronym, no checklist, no gym reps, just *can you do the lawn yet, can you do it in the wet, can you get back up the slope?, any fool can get down it.* Walking the garden's paths, purposeful movement, seeing where they take them and how they take them there, not walking between parallel bars or on a machine or staying on the spot, going somewhere, leading far away from the main building, with gravel – GRAVEL, no one can wear prosthetics on gravel, according to the rule books – but they can if they practise enough and are prepared to fall and get scuffed.

There's also long grass, wet in the rain, slippery, where they couldn't see where they were placing prosthetic feet, and fallen apples all over the ground in the ghost orchard – try watching out for those when walking. The long paths had stone edges: walk along those one prosthetic foot in front of the other, like children do with arms spread and hands flat, keep balanced as long as possible, all the way to the end, then faster. A pile of old wooden railway sleepers lying in a heap just somewhere: walk up and down on those, on and off the end into the grass and weeds. Focus, fall, roll, go back in the gym and tone up the muscles needed so no falling next time. Faster.

They needed a physio to support them as they went further and further out along the paths, and they found one in particular keeping step with them, thoughtfully, and with a Thera-Band in his pocket (all working physios stow one of those resistive latex bands somewhere). He'd been the physio at Birmingham when Mark Ormrod was extubated and in Afghanistan, and was now at Headley as complex trauma clinical lead, and he knew about choices and goals, and that the garden offered so many more of those than the gym alone. Go up the slope while being pulled backwards by the Thera-Bands, or being dragged forward, so they have to lean back and redistribute their weight and still make the joints work. Improvise with whatever is there. The gardeners have left their wheelbarrows behind this morning – so push a wheelbarrow, then a loaded wheelbarrow and then, leaning down, take a heavy spade, dig it into a pile of grass clippings, load and lift it up and turn to tip it into the wheelbarrow, and push the wheelbarrow they just loaded up, and then a lawn mower just like they'd done at home and could see now that they would do again. Almost everyone enjoyed the competition, seeing who could do what faster than all the rest, up on to big legs, weights, heavier weights, longest in the garden, weaving a racing track around the trees in the orchard and the nuttery trip, on the rotting apples, get up, go on. Get to the end first, and keep moving where the end is so the competition never ends until darkness falls and the physio, who is surprisingly forceful when he needs to be, orders them inside.

But at the end of the autumn of 2009 the gardeners came and cleared up the apples and mowed the long grass, and all the difficult things were easy again. But they didn't want to go back in the gym and sit on a boring Swiss ball, or walk up and down boring ramps in a full room where the lights were bright and unnatural and cleaning never quite managed to shift the smell left behind by human beings straining with all their might. Where they'd come to terms with what they saw in the mirror, but they didn't need to see it all the time, every step and every second, every pulse beat and every strain. Their physio found that he was frustrated too, because he wanted to push a few limits himself. He saw how the garden was making them feel really better, all of them, including him, not just more adept with their new bodies and their skills. How they stood on the lawn and laughed and planned, hands on hips, balanced. They were growing in a garden that might help everyone to flourish and discover the remnants of themselves, which had once been extraordinary and were still there, under the damage of the storm. So within one garden he conceived of another, specially and newly made to grow challenges in. He'd read *The Secret Garden* at an impressionable age, especially the part where Colin, who might have been one of Sir Robert Jones's crippled children, says to Dickon, who works in the garden: 'You said that you'd have me walking about here same as other people – and you said that you'd have me digging. I thought you were just lying to please me. This is only the first day and I've walked – and here I am digging.'[4] And because of that, I always think of the physio as Dickon; when I told him, he laughed in that way that meant he didn't really mind.

So when the physio first talked about building a special garden to meet challenges in, his patients thought it was a brilliant idea and demanded, because they are soldiers, an assault course, designed for prosthetic wearers. Good idea, he got what they were going for, but unhelpful name. So he came up with test track – like the Formula One teams have, with, as they put it, many different kinds of turns and corners. So he stood where the long main lawn rolls down from the main house at Headley, halfway down the gravel path and turn left. A patch of boring flat lawn became the test track, built in a figure of eight within an oblong enclosure. It fitted neatly into the old dividing lines of the garden's brick walls and yew hedges.

The test track was everything in the main garden that helped with walking and movement all rolled into one easily time-able course. It's still there, and if you can go to one of those open garden days they sometimes have, you'll recognise it immediately. The pathways are all different – gravel ones, cobbled ones, paved ones with insets of gravel and cobbles, a section made from split logs laid with the semicircle upwards (especially mean, this one) – and all have extra difficulties sneaked in, such as cambers, unexpected humps, slopes, uneven edges, bits sticking up, trip hazards. So not the perfect space it looks from a distance – and this was a serious problem when the contractors came to build the garden. They tried to level everything – no gradients, no humps, no edges, no cambers – but life, said the physio, isn't like that; it's not the yellow brick road without encumbrances. On the short journey round the track we need to find all the sharp edges and surprises that you find on the longer journey round life.

The track goes up and down stairs of varying height and depth to flat spaces with multi-step units, as though Mr Escher has dropped by and left one of his puzzles behind for them, up and down, keep their balance, lift their knee for a six-inch drop or a three-inch one. Life has lots of unexpected stairways, and the body needs to be ready for them, strong enough: for instance, in the pub they like, with some chairs by a fireplace that they get to up a badly lit, tight set of steps round a corner, while carrying an overfilled mug of coffee in one hand and their iPad in the other, so the banisters aren't much help. Life is about having things in both hands that can't always be put down, so they raced to the multi-step unit in the walled garden every day and practised until the light went or the surprisingly-forceful-when-he-needed-to-be physio chased them inside and off their legs.

The minute the track went down, it was full of testers. There were banisters and resting places for those at the beginning of their journey, who needed something to hold on to and somewhere to stop and gather themselves, but no one stayed on these very long. Time trials, endurance trials, like the wet grass in the orchard, doing the circuit wearing a welder's mask so their vision was occluded, learning to feel what they walked on through their foot units and their titanium joints, trusting their own steps. That really woke up their central nervous system. Texture, substance, felt at the knees, not at the toes. Even on rainy days, never mind that the prosthetic workshop lot said *don't get the £20,000 microprocessor wet* because the track was even more difficult when it was slippery – even more real. In the heavy snow of 2010, when all the garden was covered and white, out they went with the physio, who suggested snowball fights, provided they bent down and crumped the snowballs together without help and then hurled them and dodged the ones hurled back at them. (The medical term for this process is the rehabilitation of ballistic upper limb muscle power.) Those snowballs, thrown at Headley in 2010, were small frozen miracles of what humans can do when they really try. Snow marking out new lines on the walls, making the garden something completely different – as magical as the freezing of the Thames – and the sound of laughter in the cold.

Next stop along the pathway: the real world beyond the walls. If they'd shown they could take the worst of circuiting the test track and still remain upright, and they weren't having anything but minor niggles with their socket, easily fixed by the prosthetics workshop, then it was off to London for hard-core long legs boot camp. There are some things not even the walled garden at its best can prepare them for: mainly, crowds. In crowds they will inevitably be jostled, and it can all be too much. Wearing shorts can help, because people see their pros-thetics and they adjust, but not in the crowds flowing over city bridges and on busy shopping streets, heads down, headphones in, looking at screens, moving fast and focused, intolerant, used to bumping and being bumped.

So when they were ready, a whole group of them led by the physio took a train to Waterloo Station, through electronic ticket barriers, down to the tube, flowing with the crowds, escalators with their metal-teethed steps, out for the entire day, no chance of slipping back to their room at Headley to switch to stubbies or back in the chair. Embankment tube by the river, over the footbridge where the wind suddenly gusted hard over the water, through the crowds, and past the sudden distrac-tion of the bad busker, and down a really tricky set of stairs to the skateboard park claimed from a concrete undercroft on the South Bank.[5] They have ramps there too, and ledges and banks and sets of stairs, and on boot camp afternoons they have their own set of Headley patients using them while the board-ers stand back in amazement. And then a riverboat, getting on a riverboat from the bankside, sailing and standing on a deck watching the city go by but the wind making the water choppy, and then Tower Bridge, where there were plenty of steps and stairs, and back to Headley in the evening. A whole day without the chair, in the real world, and every day after that meant time at their full height, balance, strength.

It was thought, before 2009, that people who had both their

legs amputated at the thigh (bilateral transfemorals, which gets shortened to bi-lats) would never walk, no matter who they were or why it happened. Most of the physios and prosthetists who went to Headley were told this when they trained at college. There might be one or two exceptions, but not enough to count. Bilateral transfemoral amputees never walk. One day there was a fire alarm at Headley, and everyone had to exit the house quickly and assemble in the gym until the all-clear sounded. One of the prosthetists who had been told this at college looked across the gym and saw four bilateral trans-femoral amputees standing on their legs, chatting, laughing, waiting to go back to work. Bilateral transfemoral amputees are limited by their own recovery and the technology of prosthetics, that's all. Much remains to be done by others, but ask what you like of them, and they will get up and do it.

20

Sockets and Stumps and Pain

THEY DO IT UNTIL SUDDENLY THEY CAN'T, in the months during and after Headley, and now, years later. No matter how fit, or how far they have travelled, no matter how good it has been, every day the sockets and stumps found a way to remind them that it will never be all good, all improvement. Tweak medication, rest, ice bath maybe, massage and physio directly on the stump, and slowly things calm down. But not always. And this is what happens to everyone who has left part of themselves behind in Afghanistan, eventually. Where they find themselves is not necessarily, despite the work and the questions and the garden, a very hopeful place. A hard question: why do prosthetic limbs have the least chance of matching the performance of the human body?

For a start, everything anyone can think of can go wrong. Sometimes, many times, a problem with socket fit for no particular reason means something is going wrong deep inside the stump, changing its shape from within, and this never happens without a very great deal of pain. It can be almost anything. The bone end, neatly clipped and tidied up, shifting within the muscle mass. Bones malform, and bone grows in tissue that wasn't even bone in the first place (more about that in the next part). Or the muscle mass can shrink back, so physios come back and work to stretch them out again. Neuromas: nerves tidied away so carefully at Birmingham swell or develop growths that are pressed upon by the bones or muscles or ulcers or scarring or movement or shifts in weight. Nerves in the flaps change and squirm, and in a matter of days they can turn the most relaxed and confident patient into a sleep-deprived, ghost-faced bundle of pain, wincing at the slightest touch, back up on the pain ladder, all the way to the top: severe pain, uncontrollable, only the strongest drugs can touch it. The healing process itself can cause what seem like endless problems months and months after the first twenty-four days, when they have started to dare to ask what next. Then scarring skin at the stump shrinking back or, worse, galloping away with itself, creating lumps and bumps and misshapes that mean it was almost not worth bothering casting a socket in the first place.

Even if all that is going well, physio, rehab, walking, balancing, falling, just not being in a chair, all of this puts pressure on muscles that they have to learn to adapt to or strain and fail. Ulceration happens when a strained muscle can no longer recover, so the muscle tissue starts to break down instead of mend, closing off capillaries, shutting off blood flow not all the way to point zero but a little death nonetheless: no blood, no oxygen, no nutrients, no energy, so the muscle and surrounding deep soft tissues start to atrophy. And no matter how many laps of the test track they've done, what got them to Headley in the first place has wrecked their immune system, so infection finds those little patches of them that have begun to buckle under strain and take hold. But this all takes time. These pressure ulcers happen first without pain, while they are out in the garden, on the train to London, beating someone at something and going to bed happy. Then pain, and, last of all, the injury happening on the inside spreads and spreads and is finally visible on the outside, on their skin, tender to the touch but deeply damaged all the way through.

There's a new bit of kit, a hand-held scanner that can detect the deep tissue damage early before it makes it to the outside, but this isn't a rehab bit of kit, it's hospital kit, because pressure ulcers are usually found on ill people, who can't move, stuck in bed – bed sores are pressure ulcers – who have to be moved by other people. Stump ulcers happen to people trying every waking moment of every day to be moving, faster and better, months after they have left Headley and gone home to their new lives. Treatment is off the legs, even for small ulcers, and special creams and dressings. But the big ones may need debriding or surgery, so back to the past, back in their chair, almost back to Bastion in their stress levels, and almost certainly going back to Birmingham for more surgery.

The plastic surgeon got used to seeing people months or even years after he had first seen them, for a second, late stage of reconstruction, cutting away even more of what had been so carefully saved and then worked on at Headley. All of the hard work wasted, back on the table, pushing the stump higher, more difficult to find skin and muscle for flaps. De-gloving the stump: sometimes the surgeons end up redoing the entire envelope of soft tissue around the amputation site from scratch. And they know that they will be seeing the same patients for four or five years – same problems, stump and socket, in or out of the army, and we still don't know for how long this will go on.[1] And the surgeons can tell immediately the operation begins that these are patients for whom the deal has been done, who are years after their original casualty physiologically different from everyone else who passes through their hands. Difficult cases, difficult questions: has it all been worth it? Do I have to go through all that again? Will I ever be out of this chair? Back to square one, back to Headley, start again. Square one seems huge the second time they land on it, but the physios are there, and they haven't forgotten and they know what it is to start again. So a new socket, roll on the sock, up to a stand.

Back in 1918 pain was almost inevitable. One senior orthopaedic surgeon in desperation wrote after the First World War that he had a patient whose prosthetic had fitted beautifully and worked beautifully, and so he had emigrated to the West Indies to begin a new life farming a plantation there (fresh air worked as well then as it does now).[2] But then the pain had come back, so bad he could do nothing but take his savings and use them to pay his way back to Britain, back to the surgeon to see what he could do about it. And what he could do about it was very little, except perhaps to operate again and, when that failed, give the patient a list of drugs for him to take. Locomotor systems failing, not because of mechanical failure, because that was mostly fixable, but because of pain. Pain followed the casualties of the First World War home, along the train tracks, into the hospitals, paused for breath and then back again, months after everyone thought the new system was starting to work. Pain left patients healed but not cured, knocked them off their new delicate and complicated artificial limbs, warped and twisted the stumps so they no longer fitted the sockets made for them.[3] Disability was the condition, but pain was the aftermath that everyone dreaded.

In the twenty-first century, whether a military or civilian sufferer, 'post-amputation pain remains an extremely challenging pain condition to treat', according to one of the leading pain journals in the world.[4] Research done at Headley in the last year of the war in Afghanistan found that at least 65 per cent of their patients suffered from pain in their stumps severe enough for them to classify it as treatment failure.[5] Treatment failure meant back to the multidisciplinary team meeting and probably adjustments to meds, if there was no other obvious reason for the pain, and then hope.

It is much the same thing with the phantoms their patients brought with them from the wards at Birmingham, where the nurses had tried to help. At Headley half of amputee patients suffered from phantom limb pain bad enough to be distressing. At Headley treatment for phantom limb pain was about everything but changing meds. 'The patient', wrote the physio and the pain consultant, 'has to understand that [meds] are not going to remove all pain. Indeed, the degree of pain relief [...] is almost irrelevant.'[6] So, in addition to irrelevant meds, patients were encouraged to try physical therapies: looking at their stumps in mirrors, looking at themselves using their prosthetics in mirrors, helping their own brain to adjust, acupuncture, special exercises. Same principle as at Birmingham, giving the patient a measure of control. That helps, a little, hopefully, but there is no research to support it all so far.

These numbers are almost exactly the same as those for the amputee cohort in the First World War. This means that, over a century, we have made no further progress in treating chronic, life-wrecking pain in military amputees.[7] A century, and a cohort of 41,000, with nothing to show for it – not just for soldiers but for everyone whose lives are wracked by pain today. This is what happens when specialist centres and networks are closed down, and the cohort, the knowledge and expertise are scattered and unable to consolidate what they learned to make progress not only for their military patients but beyond. This is the sort of thing I go on about in meetings. A century wasted, and it can't be allowed to happen again. The pain consultant, who conceived the system used in Afghanistan of pain care from point of wounding, hopes that 'what occurs here must link with what has gone before and what will follow.'[8] The continuum of pain care must go beyond Headley, because the terms of the deal done for their lives demand it. The consultant hopes that there will be some way of having a thirty-year, 13,000-mile pain service for every military patient he ever saw, and there are some reasons for him to be hopeful. But not many, and hope is not a tactic.[9]

21

PTSD (Trauma Reaction)

IN THE PUBLIC MIND one particular condition is synonymous with all wars – not just the wars in Afghanistan – and it doesn't have anything to do with physical wounding. Instead, the focus is on the psychological stress that military personnel find themselves experiencing, which is commonly called Post-Traumatic Stress Disorder. PTSD is an acronym that has come to stand for a range of symptoms that are caused as a result of experiencing trauma, including memory loss, cognitive problems, insomnia, anxiety and depression. The stuff of novels, poetry and nightmares. A range of symptoms with a range of consequences, including the destruction of families, addiction, utter soul-destroying hopelessness, suicide. When patients at Headley suffered periods of sorrow or anxiety or depression during their treatment, the response from outside was often, *Oh have you got PTSD?* A hard question, and really not a very helpful one. So much more was going on in every aspect of their lives where their physical and psychological experiences were interlinked. They might have PTSD, and for those that are suffering from acute symptoms there is a dedicated mental health unit at Headley to which they can be referred. But for most, a single PTSD diagnosis was not even relevant.

The material in this chapter is drawn from what I was told by the physio and by other physios and members of the multidisciplinary teams working with patients at Headley.

Unexpected survivors had unexpected and complex consequences of their survivorship. Rehabilitation was never just going to be about their new physical selves, but their team members had very little to go on to guide them beyond the gym. When they spoke of it among themselves, they called it, very simply, the 'trauma reaction', and they meant all those things that weren't about joints or muscles or stumps or sockets. There were no clinical trials or questionnaires, just their own therapeutic instincts and those are what they told me about, and the results as they saw them. I think those instincts were right (unsurprisingly), and I think they have much to contribute to broader discussions of PTSD, but for the moment we stay at Headley and the reasons why this chapter should really be called 'Trauma Reaction'.

Think of PTSD as a single layer among many of the things that can settle on the human brain as a consequence of traumatic injury. It's like the illustrations in geography textbooks, of rock layers – stratigraphy – where one has to distinguish between individual layers (strata) and what they layer themselves into (stratification). The separate components knitting together into a whole that is distinctive and different. Traumatic injury of any kind wraps the brain in layers, each of which requires distinct treatment, some quite different from the others, but the layers can bleed into each other, making all their effects worse. Any treatment must be for both the layers and their interaction. The medical term is 'complex co-morbidity', and there is so much about it that we don't yet understand, but we are starting to (more about that later).

At Headley a good place to start sorting out the layers was by the side of the patients who stared in the mirrors, trying to make out what their new selves were. The team saw that this part of the trauma reaction was about uncertainty, and much of it was about grief. Their patients grieved for the lost parts of themselves, and the lost friends and comrades who had not made it this far. Because they were specialists in rehab, the team also knew, better than anyone else, what pain does to a recovering human's body and how it affects a mind already carrying layers of damage. Three separate layers just here to distinguish and make sense of: loss of self, grief, pain. Settling round the brain, interacting, each making the other worse. Psychological and physical, all at the same time.

Recognising these reactions to trauma led the teams to understand in more general terms how not everyone in the buildings around them was quite ready to come outside into the bright light and open air. That they didn't all plan their day around competitions where the worst conceivable outcome for the loser was being called crap-hat till bedtime. Where moving into the wider, sometimes noisy, spaces of the garden was a frightening step, so the best thing would be to move from one known space to another, still the garden but different, and where other things might be done with different remnants, with the selves every bit as shattered as the bones and muscles.

For this the physio remembered that there was a greenhouse, built with the original house for plants that don't do well in adverse circumstances such as frost and heavy rain, that need warmth and special care. He had the greenhouse rebuilt and every pane of glass restored by contractors from the local water company, who had also worked on the test track. Inside it's just like any other greenhouse, provided your greenhouse standard is quite grand. It's warm and slightly humid and light, but there is green lichen on the glass panes and mud splashes from when it rains, so the brightness is softened. The smell is different from anywhere else, damp and mossy, things growing, leaf by leaf gradually unfurling in the light and warmth.

There's a particular pot that's been there for several years, and when the physio goes into the greenhouse, he looks for it (and so do I). It's a very average-looking red chilli plant, except that, like the greenhouse it grows in, there's nothing average about it because it was the very first plant in the garden at Headley raised entirely by a patient from seed. Suffering a severe trauma reaction, he had got as far as the greenhouse, and pushed inside its warmth and light as if one more moment spent outside would crush him, and only the greenhouse offered shelter. He was shown round, which didn't take long, and then given the chilli seeds and a small black plastic flowerpot with compost in it. Push the seeds in – it doesn't matter if this isn't the sort of thing they've done before – little bit of water, put it on the shelf, come back tomorrow and see if anything has happened. Come back tomorrow. And soon delicate seedlings poke through the compost, the first leaves and then branches, and then it will need re-potting, and don't worry, we've got plenty of bigger ones, and then, like bright red miracles, chillies. Which they can take off and chop up and put on their curry. And they keep coming and the plant keeps growing, even on bad days, when the rain clouds darken the sky and standing up to work at the bench is a struggle, and they wonder if it will ever be over. The chilli plant is still there, about the size of a small shrub (and it has a whole cohort of other chilli plants, in rainbow colours from yellow to purple), with sturdy, thick branches and regular harvests of big chillies, a couple of inches long but hot as you like.

Patients came out of the greenhouse nourished and better. Standing at the planting tables they had been able to think quietly about themselves, as their hands worked, and their fingers, which trembled with the strain during the day, pushed tender seedlings down into compost, and then watered them carefully so nothing spilled over the edge with the life in it that was now theirs. A small space, sunlit and warm, where they could be immersed. Whatever they had expected to find at Headley, it hadn't been this. As more of them came to the space, more pots appeared on the low walls outside, not just chillies but other things, herbs and flowers, lavender, geranium, bay, rosemary, so when they came out of the greenhouse to sit in the sunshine and just think (and that was progress), they could touch the leaves and smell the aromatics on their fingertips – fingertips that shook a little less and, on very good days, not at all. And then everything else became a little easier. Less pain, less stress, fewer trigger points that bought back the wounding or the war, a little more physio, a few more steps forward, slow and careful, balance, learning not to fall. On one of the days I visited the garden, a patient who showed me a chilli plant he had grown told me that from now on he was going to work outside, that he and his family had bought a smallholding and that that would be their lives after his discharge from the army, although I don't know how those plans have worked out.

Greenhouse and test track, separated by one of Headley's original gravelled garden paths. Still not quite there, thought the physio. Still too separate, little worlds of their own. Headley was about tackling the whole person's rehabilitation, and recognising that a good day on the test track can suddenly be a bad day of pain and memories and grieving. The walled garden at Headley should be a whole world, with above it only sky, so how to layer the two into one? At rest the test track, with no soldiers hurling themselves round it, looked almost like a conventional garden, with steps and paths and decking, and spaces between the challenges that could easily be turned into flower beds. That was beyond the skill of the physio, but then Scott Meenagh, who had some very mixed days, said, 'My dad's a gardener', and the physio remembered the quiet man who watched them intently as they worked, sitting on the wall among the flower pots, and how comfortable he seemed there. And so Thomas Meenagh got up off the wall and joined his son and his friends and physio in the garden, and the remnants became finally a new whole. Not just a test track, and a path and a greenhouse on the other side. A garden within the original garden, and with all its power.

Along with funding (and ambitions to win a medal at the Chelsea Flower Show), Headley Court had a brief for the new garden. It had to be easily maintained, preferably by patients, because those wheelbarrows had shown that gardening was good for them, linked them with the life beyond, maybe even a new job that was still hard work and outside, but not soldiering. It had to be a garden for all seasons, with colour, texture and structure that provided interest all year round; plus microprocessors were waterproof now, so there would be no keeping anyone out, even – especially – when it snowed.

Thomas Meenagh wanted to give them much more than the brief. He had seen his son's exhilaration at his achievements on the test track, but he also knew that there was a cost to knowing that those new feet that would never feel grass between their toes in any garden ever again. He wanted somewhere to find calm and return it to his son's soul, the calm missing since 25 January and the third explosion along the dusty track. So he sought to create a place that would ease all the griefs of those who came to the garden, that allowed rest and contemplation by everyone who came to Headley, staff, patients and all the family like him, who watched sitting on the side line walls.

Thomas Meenagh chose plants that provided strong, solid structural frames at the heart of the new beds layered into the test track garden.[1] Within the frames were plants that produced an abundance of blossom: petals flying off in the wind that could be gathered up and bagged to make confetti for the weddings that happened, better late than never, to patients who came straight back to Headley for more work after the honeymoon was over. There were plants whose flowers and leaves smelled as good as they looked, in the air or on the fingertips, a different way to feel the garden now that toes could not. Plants where families could give bored children a leaf to nibble on so they could find out what herbs taste like, something to talk about while their hearts were otherwise breaking. Something to share with other family groups; 'one touch of nature makes the whole world kin.'[2] Plants that were beautiful when it rained, silver drops of water hanging from their foliage. In autumn plants that make catkins, and plants whose leaves burst fiery red, suddenly but gloriously. Plants that elegantly framed winter with frosted stems, seed heads, feathery, silvered leaves, something to look for from the windows of the house, when even the boldest preferred the warmth.

A garden for all seasons. Seasons aren't simply months and

mean temperatures; they also represent different occasions, moods, circumstances and times in the lives of human beings.[3] Trauma reactions – the layers building in a human mind that will settle and thicken and limit unless someone gently smooths them away. Thomas Meenagh understood this, as the physios had done, so the garden he built for his son and all the families at Headley sought out meaning beyond the annual planting cycles and five human senses. Above all, as he watched his son he came to understand that, even though he was rebuilding, he was also grieving deeply. Scott wore then, and wears to this day, a wristband with the name of his comrade who died at his point of wounding back in January 2011. At Headley he grieved for him as well as for his own lost self, for the whole that was gone . Thomas Meenagh saw that his son's life journey was to be made on his new legs but also through the layers inside his head, and there were bumps, and adverse cambers and gravel that he had to make his way over, and that this was hard.

Thomas Meenagh had his gardening students working with him, and as he discussed the project with them, one pointed out to him that there were different stages of bereavement and that perhaps they could reflect those in their planting.[4] Layers within layers. So in each new bed in the garden were plants that had seasonal interest, stimulated the five human senses and represented the six stages of bereavement. Because the father knew that the son sometimes had good days and bad days, and that these were muddled around, not progressive, he put plants representing different stages next to each other in groups, light and dark, bright and black, all on the same day, in the same life.

Denial: black/deep purple
Anger: red
Bargaining: purple/blue
Depression: orange
Acceptance: yellow
Peace: white/green

By now there were many physios and horticultural therapists who worked in the gardens and stood by the side of those in the greenhouse and showed them how to pot things up. So he went to them and told them how the system of plants and colours and stages worked, so they would have another way to start conversations, to help give form to feelings that seemed chaotic, helping patients and family and medics understand and accompany each other along the way.

The garden grew, and a miniature version of it won a bronze medal at Chelsea. The orchard was restored (but not the poor old inappropriately named nuttery). Yard by yard more beds were added, for flowers and vegetables, and pots sprouted on every low wall. Mowing, watering, tending (although Thomas Meenagh had thoughtfully put a permeable membrane over the soil of his planted areas and crushed slate and marble chippings to suppress weeds). Chickens too, in a new area fenced off just alongside the test track. According to the physio, a lot can be understood about a person's recovery by the way they handle a chicken. So Headley's newest population is a brood of calmly tolerant hens. Once patients have worked in the greenhouse and nurtured a plant in a little black plastic pot, then they may be ready to go outside, and then they are handed a chicken. If they are able to shift their attention to the slightly grumpy warm bundle of feathers in their arms, if they try to make it comfortable, look it in its beady eye, and then set it down gently back in the pen, then they are moving on, moving outside themselves. It's engagement, of a kind that they can manage when other kinds seem infinitely difficult, but it leads on to more.[5] So they come back to feed the chickens, and make sure they are hutched at night, and collect their eggs for the kitchen. Warm soil, warm eggs – things they have carefully and thoughtfully found or made, and that mean something.[6]

The garden had become a space where the physio could dream and build solutions, as if the creativity that made an entire sundial out of hedges and all the other joyful eccentricities of the place came back and settled on him. Or perhaps it was the fresh air. Either way, if he'd been told years before that this was what he would have ended up with, he would never have started the project, but now no one can imagine Headley without the garden, and it is the first thing visitors are shown round on tours. There were times when perhaps a little too much fresh air made him a little too creative. He suggested a herd of micropigs penned into the orchard, to eat the windfalls and grass, and so that people could try their hand at small animal husbandry, but micropigs are beyond the scope of even the most enlightened military medical authority, so it's still only chickens. But everyone acknowledges their special chicken powers because when occasionally a Surrey fox sweeps in for a massacre, they are swiftly replaced, therapists driving through the night to collect duplicates from obliging farmers and breeders.

But none of this is really accidental, and this goes beyond the new kinds of horticultural or animal therapy to something deeper, even more reparative. There's (guess what) a special scientific name for the instinctive human need to connect with other living things and systems, not just themselves: biophilia. Chickens and chilli plants, newly laid warm eggs in a warm human hand: biophilia. Coming to understand ourselves as we understand other organisms, watching them grow as we grow, taking care of them as we learn to care for ourselves: biophilia. Naturalists and biologists are specialists in biophilia, but all they really do is make a living from an instinct that all humans have. We evolved in intimate contact with the natural environment, and when we need to regroup, going back into a place of growing life helps us re-evolve, rediscover what we were, even if the forest is eons gone and the place we walk in is a walled garden, newly planted.[7] In nature things grow through the layers, finding the smallest cracks from dry clay to old soil through the semi-permeable membrane. Life, as someone once said in a dinosaur film, will find a way.[8]

In the garden Scott Meenagh understood, as he came to the low points in his new life, that, although some people at

Headley needed to go all the way to the psych unit hidden behind the hedges for a formal mental health session, he was not one of them. Talking was best for him, with someone at his side, walking with him over the low point, around the corner, out of the dark. Side-by-side therapy for trauma reaction. Mark Ormrod's girlfriend, sitting at his side on the floor leaning up against the sofa. The horticultural therapist at the side of a patient working on the tables in the greenhouse, explaining renewal, softening pain. Physios walking alongside a patient down pathways into cool shade, even though the timetable said that during that hour they should be doing cardiovascular fitness, but instead doing a different version of the session on improving confidence on challenging terrain. Difficult to formalise and not for everyone, but for most, and best done with something beautiful to look at or useful to do at the same time. Smoothing out some of the layers together, never possible to get them all gone completely, but fewer layers, so less complicated later on (hopefully).

*

I didn't expect to spend most of a chapter on rehabilitation writing about a garden, but the power of the place astounded me, and it still does. Gyms and prosthetic workshops and treatment rooms have complex things going on in them, but if we understand what happened in the garden, then we understand everything. There are plenty of articles that list the benefits of horticulture on the sick, and they are listed in this note.[9] There are histories of gardens in hospitals, particularly those created by superstar designers in the twenty-first century.[10] But Headley doesn't quite fit neatly into the category of hospital garden or horticultural therapy site – it is both and more. It is, borrowing the words of the team members who created it, a reaction to trauma. It's a defiant garden on a much larger scale than that in the terracotta pots in a corner of Camp Bastion, but it is based on some of the same principles. A defiant garden is one that is created in response to a challenge, that provides mechanisms of human survival, and that provides evidence for human creativity and resilience in extreme circumstances.[11] The deal for life may have been done, its terms may have been difficult, but the garden changes the setting. No more desert, no more bright artificial hospital ward lights. Instead, somewhere to grow again, anew.

I think it may also be something to do with the fact that, unlike most hospital gardens, which are spaces hacked out of car parks or architectural blind spots, Headley is layered into an existing garden – its remnants, but still a very fine garden with deep memories dormant in its ground. Like compost dug through tired soil, layering in the new garden brought the old one back to life. The old one was connected to some of the earliest human thinking about making gardens and what they can be used for. The oldest gardens were in monasteries, places in which to heal and to contemplate, and most of them looked like Headley. They were full of pathways and resting places, and were bounded by high, strong walls – not to enclose or imprison but to focus the mind, shield it from too much reality, but with a gate for when suitable strength had been generated. At Headley only the sky above is unbounded – infinite and eternal.[12]

Looking up into its grey or its rain or, best of all, its blue is a timeless human impulse, seeking contemplation, comfort, healing from places of horror and pain. On the Western Front during the First World War men stuck in bloody mud looked up when the sun came out and the gun smoke cleared. Stretcher-bearers trawling with their loads through deep dark trenches were grateful for any sliver of sky they could see above them. At night doctors and soldiers on both sides stood on something high (and safe) and picked out constellations of stars in the night sky, using charts sent to them from home. At a remarkable hospital working with the shell-shocked come home from that war a theory of colour therapy was developed, where ceilings were painted firmament blue so that those not yet ready for the journey to the outside could begin to contemplate it.[13] (Thomas Meenagh would be pleased to see that the walls were yellow – acceptance – and the woodwork picked out in green – peace – although the original intention was to replicate feelings associated with spring.) All the same sky, look up at it and begin to heal.

It is almost as if the walled garden at Headley willed itself into being because of the great human need that emanated from the house along the paths and lawns (don't tell any of the scientists I work with that I wrote that). Perhaps its power came from the group of people that gathered there at exactly the right time to make it: patients, their physio and a father, the gardener. Perhaps the greatest power of all is this: it works even though the visitor can never quite get away from the world of the twenty-first century, wherever they go in the garden. Beyond the walls are busy roads and motorways, and the sound of traffic is constant, like a noise made by a powerful waterfall in the distance, running day and night. So the garden can never be a total refuge, total escape, total shelter, and it does what it can, which isn't by any means everything. No one can stay absent in it for ever, and when they tune in, they can hear the sounds of the real world beyond, to which they will eventually return.

PART THREE

BEYOND

'Good luck for your onward
journey and beyond.'

MERT paramedic, in Scott Meenagh's
patient diary, 25 January 2011

22

The Engineer: Dave Henson

And then I actually lost my legs …

Dave Henson, interview in the sound archives of the National Army Museum

Dave – Everyone is thinking about you.

Can I have your Timberlands?

Is it too early …?

Entry in Dave Henson's patient diary, 2225 hrs, 13 February 2011

MORE THAN ANYONE ELSE in this book, Dave Henson understands every single step on the journey back from the first
moments of survival on into the future of living fully as a
double amputee. His grandfather had served in the RAF in
the Second World War. He'd been a radar operator, and the
constant strain of staring at one of the early video screens in
dim light for hours on end had ruined his sight. So Dave knew
from an early age that military service could have its costs, that
one rarely came without the other, and just in case he hadn't
registered it growing up, his grandfather made sure he knew
that this was why he had reservations about him joining the
army but at the same time, at the end of the conversation, how
proud he was of his grandson.

Dave had registered everything, and not just in a very
general way but quite specifically, about the war he would

go to. He'd been thinking about injury even before, during his engineering undergraduate degree, where his final-year project was to build an access mechanism for getting people in wheelchairs in and out of go-karts. He'd spent a fair bit of time in a wheelchair, to understand how it felt and what the constraints were. So when he went to Afghanistan as a Royal Engineer working as part of the Counter-IED Task Force, he was, in the strangest and most thoughtful way possible, ready.

> I knew the risks that were associated with it. I'd spent time adjusting before to the possibility of not having any legs when I came back so before I went on tour I made sure I'd climbed a mountain so I could tick that box off my To Do list just in case it happened, and then I actually lost my legs so I was aware of the possibility and that helped a lot. All the guys seemed to make jokes about losing their legs before they go but I think I really knew it was a possibility and had accepted it before I went so I came back and I had an idea of what it would take to get on with things. And then you just crack on, I guess.

There are simpler reasons too why Dave remembers every step of his journey. He was, unusually, awake for most of them. On Sunday 13 February 2011 he was leading a patrol into two compounds previously used by the enemy as firing positions, and this usually meant IEDs had been left behind for the next occupants to discover. They were an experienced team by now, with over twenty IEDs found and disabled. They cleared one compound: nothing. Then into the second: something. Weight placed on to a trigger, heartbeat thuds under the beaten sand floor, Dave thrown up into the air, and then falling forward, landing on his head, his face on the ground. No blue sky bright above him, or seconds to reflect. Just pain and trying to right himself, to sit up, to use his hands – gloved, but he'd cut the tips off so his fingers were already scratched and bleeding from the day's earlier work – to lift his weight and drag it so he could lean up against a wall, backing away from whatever was left of the device and the sight of what it had done to him, as if it could be left behind under the settling dust with all the other debris. He didn't recognise what came with him as he moved, what he was dragging, and he began to scream even as the echo of the blast died.

His men got to him immediately. He knew what to do: lots of drills. He knew because he'd made them do them, over and over again. There were a few raised voices, to get him to stop screaming, as they gathered round him and started to work. So he stopped. He breathed a few times, and started to give instructions instead, that they should get the radio, get the camera to take a picture of the site of the explosion for future reference (he uses the picture of the hole in presentations), but he saw that they were doing everything before he said it, calling down MERT, reading out the 9-Liner, a T1, one of their own, needing a stretcher, no particular concerns about the safety of the landing site outside the compound walls, and someone was taking a picture of the small crater and its consequences. He calmed himself and looked again at his shredded legs and realised as he dared to scan down that he could see to the end of his limbs. That his boots were still on his feet and what was left of his legs was just about attached to his body, but the engineer in him knew they weren't viable as walking implements any more. And then he had the bottle of water one of his lads handed him, and because he smoked, he had a cigarette, and by the time he had finished it and a few others, and stubbed them out in the bloody sand, they'd finished working on him, and the helicopter was landing, and MERT crew were bursting out of the back, heading for him.

He was still awake and not yet crashing, but had lost a lot of blood, so the medics bent over him got the lines in, and because he still wasn't crashing or needing intubating, the helicopter became a pre-operative ward, prepping him at a steady pace for surgery, giving him the anaesthetic in advance, so that thirty-seven minutes after the blast he would be on the table in the operating theatre at Bastion. A double amputation, right one off above the knee, left one through the knee. Then he was back on the ward, and the nurses started his patient diary:

> I was your nurse today at Camp Bastion. This morning when I came on shift I woke you up. You are doing really well. Well enough to moan about having a cigarette. When your CO turned up we took you outside in the sunshine for a smoke and you seemed really happy with that. Of all the patients I have cared for you have the most visitors so you sound like a popular guy. Good luck with your rehab. Don't lose that lovely spirit on this road to recovery.

He had to wait longer than normal for the CCAST flight to bring him home, so Dave's nurse and CO wheeled his bed outside the ward so he could smoke. His new stumps were examined by the hand surgeon, with the Doe a Deer bleep, and who remembers conducting a ward round outside during Dave's fag breaks and that this wasn't standard NHS practice. Dave remembered studying the rest of the camp from where he lay in his hospital bed outside and being impressed with how it had developed.

In 2006, as a student, he'd been part of an army engineering team that planned and drilled the original four bore holes for the water essential to the camp's establishment. He hadn't actually gone to what was becoming Bastion, he'd been too junior for that, but he'd done all the paperwork they needed back in the UK, and made the noticeboards that went up for the equipment and read the reports that came back of what the bore holes were drilling into. Dust and fines on the top, plenty of water 150 metres down, in a hard coral aquifer that drained fresh water from the snowmelt of the Hindu Kush mountain range into the camp in the middle of the desert, so there'd be no more problems with supply lines. Enough for 100,000 litres to be pumped up a day: about half used for drinking and the rest for dampening down the dust and fines, and for the fire engines, one of which always waited by the MERT landing site. So when he arrived he could actually see what his team had achieved, and he always admired anything to do with the water he had helped to bring to the surface: things like the water purification and bottling plant, which were kept as clean as the hospital and produced stacked pallets' worth of bottled drinking water every hour.

More visitors. Dave's unit had come back to Bastion during the day of his wounding, so they all made their way to the field hospital and braced themselves for what they would find, and fought for the pen so they could write in his patient diary (three volumes in the end, the only multi-volume diary produced in the whole Afghan campaign, from what I've found so far), and tried not to let him see what they were feeling when they looked at him. They had brought his belongings with them, so he could take them home. Like all soldiers, Dave had been shopping before coming out to Afghanistan, and he hadn't worn much of it before he was injured.

One of the first to visit him found him still sleeping from the anaesthetic. He sat by the pile of belongings he had brought and was able to write the difficult thing he might otherwise have had to say face to face. Dave had no more need of the trousers he had bought on leave; it would be shorts from now on.

> Just arrived and got a chance to speak to the MERT dr. Apparently you were hard to shut up LOL. He said the boys did an awesome job treating you, all that content training by you paid off and the boys came through. Couldn't find any shorts when getting your things together so you've got mine instead – hope they fit as I'm a short arse.

Another friend was less reticent about tackling the subject of Dave's most recent purchases. They all had heavy-duty desert boots to work in, but Dave had brought another brand-new pair out with him as well, to wear back in camp off-duty, a bit flashier than the work ones. His were top-of-the-range, waterproof, seam-sealed, insulated, anti-fatigue midsole, leather-covered foot-bed for premium feel and optimum comfort, with a padded collar that eases ankle pressure and, in a nod to ecological considerations, long durable laces made of 100 per cent recycled plastic bottles. ('Disco shoes' is the technical military term.) They had cost a fortune, and he had hardly worn them.

> Dave. Big Love!!! Everyone is thinking about you. Can I have your Timberlands? Is it too early?

And then they all came, one by one, his unit. The young men who had stood and watched alongside him at the patrol base, there to fight, not to write, and now fighting for the pen, words streaming on to the page: old-fashioned for the generation used to keyboards and textspeak, but somehow, in this place, the right thing to do.

> Alright Troopy [Dave's nickname], don't know where to start. Before I do you will have to excuse my Johnny age 3 handwriting and spelling. When I found out, I couldn't quite believe what had happened. [We] are a bulletproof lot but when I came in to see you and saw you in the bed it sunk in. The doc looking after you at the time told us of your progress which put my mind at ease a bit …

Then CCAST arrived to take him home. He was flying back with another Critical Care patient, and as they were being wheeled out to the Globemaster, the other patient crashed, trauma medics swarming over him, reviving him three times before they got a stable heartbeat. Dave could do nothing but watch, adding his voice to those calling out numbers and vital signs, encouraging him to hold on, hold on. He did, so they moved off again, both patients on board.

As the hours and miles flew by, Dave dozed, naturally, and woke and got to know the team who stood alongside him working to keep him stable. He wasn't intubated, so he could talk and eat; it was unusual for them to have a patient to talk to against the background noise and they enjoyed it. They gave him a pair of ear defenders, but he doesn't remember the noise as being particularly bad. There were one or two quiet jokes about CCAST's ability to smuggle contraband. Dave had his cigarette cartons packed in his luggage, and he wouldn't have to pay the duty on them when he got back to the UK. They shared things with him, not just conversation, grateful for a living voice and laughter from the human under the straps.

> David, so here we are, I reckon halfway home, some-where in the sky. I'm one of the anaesthetic CCAST doctors; we have the honour of making sure you get back safe to the UK. You have been a stoical and determined patient – I hope this continues during the weeks ahead. Can't believe I let you have my green Starburst – it's my favourite too.

And then home. Less wakefulness at Birmingham. No bone infection, but plenty of pain and shrapnel wounds in his back-side that wouldn't heal. His weight dropped, muscle mass disappearing, weakness. More operations, weeks of pain, and deepening fug from painkillers, not much memory of visit-ors. Gradually he recovered. More days wakeful than dopey, getting nurses to wheel him out for a cigarette, just as he had at Bastion, making the Military Matron change ward policy just for him – no real cigarettes allowed on Critical Care but e-cigarettes OK for now (they aren't any more).

Slowly he was becoming an engineer again, looking back down at where his legs no longer were, as brave every time as the first time he did it, braced up against the mud wall. A wheelchair was brought to his bedside for his trips outside. Unlike almost everyone else who lost legs in Afghanistan, he'd already been in one, knew the concept well, knew what limitations it entailed. When he grieved for his lost legs, he grieved like an engineer.

> For me with my injuries, having no knee or ankle joints, your body's natural way of correcting balance is completely shot. There is a whole chain of muscles and ligaments and nerve endings that go all the way up from your ankles, and from your knees all the way up to your pelvis and spine, which are responsible for keeping you upright. Breaking that chain from the knee and ankle, it adjusts your balance. It's not great.

And so to Headley: a socket cast, then stubbies and then walking. He lived a short drive from Headley, so as soon as he got his car with the hand controls, he told them he didn't need a room and drove home every evening – commuting to rehab. Evenings at Headley could be difficult. There was time to think, and that wasn't always a good thing, not when a person wasn't ready to do that kind of thinking. Headley was a point between two worlds – the world of the army, and the world of the civilian – and Dave wasn't quite sure where his place was any more, and finding it was going to be difficult. He needed to be in both, as much as possible, until the gulf became smaller and the movement between them easier, and then hopefully he forgot about it.

Not far along the coast from Headley, in Brighton, his grandfather was having a holiday in a place created a century before to meet the costs of military service. The St Dunstan's centre at Ovingdean was specially built in 1938 to provide respite care for those, like Dave's grandfather, with serious visual impairments. Compared with Headley, Ovingdean's gardens aren't much to speak of, but the surroundings are soft rolling downland and carefully fenced pathways leading to the seafront. Dave drove out to visit him for the first time since he lost his legs. A notice in the main hallway that told him that each of the floors was laid out in exactly the same way so their blind visitors could keep their bearings wherever they were, and to make sure he always walked on the right-hand side in the rooms and corridors – same principle as the yellow brick road at Headley. Dave followed instructions, step by step, swaying a bit on his brand new legs, but keeping to the right as instructed. His grandfather could tell as soon as he heard his voice that Dave was walking again.

Like almost everyone else at Headley, Dave had made running his primary goal for rehab. By the end of the year in which he was injured he was back in the prosthetics workshop getting fitted for his running blades. The first time he ran on the blades, his steps, one after another, faster and faster, speed for the first time in so long, speed, faster than those around him, remembering how that felt, feeling like he used to. He was good at the running, and began to think about, and then to train for, actual sports. The London Olympics were on, and the Paralympics, and he could see himself there, so he gave up smoking and started to train properly.

But running blades aren't big legs; the whole mechanism is more delicate, and if the wearer is pushing themselves, and Dave is always pushing himself, then they can fail. In a training session in 2014 one of the blades snapped and he fell, and as he fell he saw the flaw in falling-down class at Headley, because it only taught him how to fall on big legs, not blades and, as it now appeared, the skills and techniques were not necessarily transferable. As he would have done any day before 13 February 2011, he put his hands out to break his fall, and at his new fighting weight and at speed, he dislocated his shoulder, fractured his wrist and damaged his hands.

It was so true, the thing they said in falling-down class: *for every joint you lose, the more care you need to take of the ones that are left.* The injured shoulder affected his entire body, all the muscles in his core weakening because he could no longer work out properly to sustain them. So he had to wait until the injury was somewhat healed, and in the meantime he put on weight and then his socket didn't fit again, and there isn't a mulberry bush at Headley but perhaps there should be. Shoulder rehab takes much longer than leg rehab: eighteen months so far and still giving him gyp.

Today Dave sits at a desk not far from mine and taps away at his computer researching while I tap away at mine writing about his plans (and occasionally he reads what I write and says things like 'there wasn't only a hospital at Camp Bastion, there was other stuff too', which was how I found out about the bore holes). When he dreamed in the first couple of years after his injury, he dreamed of himself with legs. Now he dreams of himself with prosthetics, more and more. He's an engineer, he's well qualified to tackle the problem, he's the expert. If he can't find a way forward … he will find a way forward. And there's a solid historical precedent for him to follow.

In 1861 a young engineer injured in an unprecedentedly bloody modern war, applied his skills and brought about the greatest innovation for amputees since the invention of carpentry tools. James Hanger was a student in the engineering department of Washington College. He left to join his brothers in a Confederate regiment just in time for the first real land battle of the American Civil War, at Philippi. There were no deaths, fewer than ten casualties per side, nothing like the stinking blood-soaked overlay the conflict would become. But one of the Philippi casualties was Hanger, who had one leg shot to pieces by a Unionist cannonball, and then was captured and operated on by a Unionist surgeon. One of the very first Confederate amputees, young and incapacitated, Hanger was returned home in a prisoner exchange complete with heavy wooden peg leg.

He spent the next three months hidden away in his bedroom at home, his family thinking he was unable to come to terms with his injury. Southern men were supposed to be whole, strong, staunch defenders of their way of life, not broken and dependent. But Hanger wasn't sitting upstairs defeated by his condition; he was working in what was now mostly a workshop with a bed in the corner. And then one day his family, sitting in their parlour, heard him come downstairs. Not with the heavy, deadening thump of the wooden leg but with a different rhythm, lighter, more even. And there he was, at the bottom of the stairs, on a new leg, that he had made for himself. Not just a leg: he'd made a double jointed, articulated knee part that bent when he lifted up his thigh stump, and the leg itself was lighter, shaped like a leg, with a foot that could probably fit into a shoe when he turned his mind to that.

Hanger patented his new leg at the Confederate government's own patent office (the drawings that he made up in his bedroom still exist) and began to develop the prototype for manufacture for the casualties of battles where thousands were falling, never to return home whole.[1] Hanger went on to open factories and received approval from the eventually victorious Union government, who granted him a national patent in 1891. Driven by the needs of military amputees, Hanger's company became the largest manufacturer of prostheses in the world, as they still are. Hanger supplies and fits Mark Ormrod's three limbs. During the First World War and with the great need of its amputee cohort, Hanger went to Europe, where it was one of three American prosthetic companies to receive contracts to build workshops at the new Roehampton Hospital in London for convalescing amputees. The first Confederate amputee, on a leg of his own design, stood on the grounds of Roehampton and met casualties from the new century's war. By 1935 Hanger had become the sole military contractor to the Ministry of Pensions to provide prostheses to old and new amputees, and they maintained their position and the relationships they built then a century later.[2] One engineer in a workshop (and in case he's still wondering, I think that's where Dave belongs) can change the world, then as now.

*

Postscript. In August 2016 Dave's out of office email message changed.

> Thank you for your email. I am currently out of office in preparation for the Rio 2016 Paralympic Games. Access to email is a little sporadic in this period but I will endeavour to get back to you. I am back in on Monday 26th September.

He was back in the office on the Monday, and he brought with him the bronze medal he won in the Paralympics T42 200 m final. It's what he's holding in the picture of him in the plate section. He has a new ambition now. His daughter is getting old enough for a bike of her own. One day, quite soon probably, he'll stand behind her and watch her ride without training wheels, and centre himself to move quickly in case she falls. He'd like to be able to go out on family bike rides, but currently that is impossible for transfemoral amputees with stump and socket prosthetics. So that's what he's working on – not a bike or a new stump, but a whole system that means it will all become possible (see next section).

23

A Centre for Blast Injury Studies

I OCCASIONALLY GO DOWN to the Theoretical Physics depart-ment to ask them if the Time Machine is ready yet.[1] When it is (because so far, nothing), I'm going to ask them to send me back, not very far geographically – so presumably a rela-tively easy trip – and hopefully return just along the corridor. I want to go to the lecture by the orthopaedic surgeon who had been at the Western Front when he came to speak at Imperial College in April 1919. I'd like to know who went to his demonstration, and then perhaps take him back with me to show him that, almost a century later, two rooms along, another meeting took place, just like his, with a lantern show and cinematographic film. He could meet the group of sci-entists and medics and casualties, the people I see every day, who want to make the way into the future easier for today's wounded. One of the twenty-first-century speakers came up from Headley Court – Dave Henson's prosthetist, who was reminded of just how far they'd come by the sight of double amputees standing and talking together during the fire alarm. The physio who had seen Mark Ormrod extubated and who built the garden and the test track and the greenhouse. And a scientist who's done all the experiments to prove that their way works. That double amputees can walk, and walk well and that their step length and standing stance can be much more efficient than the literature and the out-of-date training and NHS standard indicate, and that the only limitations are prosthetic, not human.

Then I would give him the tour of the centre. He might already know about it because (and this is where having a historian in the department is handy) it turns out we've been doing blast injury research at Imperial for a century; scientists were working in laboratories even while he spoke in a lecture theatre. In 1914 one of the first volunteers for the war was Imperial's Rector, Alfred Keogh. He became Director of the Army's Medical Service and sent his closest colleague, Arthur Sloggett, out to France to observe the war and its casualties directly and to report back any particular problems.

In December 1915, after a year in which it had been made clear that artillery was going to be the main cause of casualty on the Western Front, Sloggett wrote to Keogh to ask him to initiate research into 'the effects of bomb-wounds'.[2] Imperial scientists were asked to design experiments that would produce 'accurate data as to the average velocity, size and penetrating power of bomb fragments'. To achieve this, they could apply to the Trench War Department of the War Office for samples of German bombs. They could build a special metal walled space to facilitate the collection, enumeration and examination of the fragments obtained by blowing up the German bomb samples and seeing what marks they made on the copper wall sheets. (Copper is soft and therefore especially good at this sort of thing. We still use the panels today. They have one of those names where poetry and engineering unexpectedly intersect: 'witness panels'.) Then they could use this data to design protective clothing for soldiers most likely to be in harm's way (gun crews in particular). And while they were about it, could they give some thought to a design for overalls and gauntlets capable of protecting men against the barbs of 'wire' because these losses by men 'getting hung up on wire were very serious and the moral effect was great in proportion'.

In Afghanistan throughout 2008 the physical and 'moral' effects of IEDs infesting the landscape were becoming increasingly serious for both British service personnel and their medics. As plans were made to convert the tented hospital to a hard-build, one orthopaedic surgeon had begun to think beyond the medical space and into the scientific. He had gone to Bastion as the only orthopaedic specialist in 2008, replacing one of the team who had saved Mark Ormrod. He'd asked for Bastion because he liked to find orthopaedic problems to solve, and he knew that Ormrod was an outlier, not an exception. Eventually there would be a permanent team of five orthopods at Bastion to deal with the hammering of blast injury. But for now there was just him. And a 9-Liner that told of five injured patients incoming, one of them very bad.

There had been six Afghan National Army soldiers in the vehicle that had driven over an IED, which had exploded directly beneath it. The driver had been killed outright, and four had minor injuries. Only one of the six was badly injured enough to become his patient. He was talking, so through a Terp he could tell the medical team that his vehicle had blown up, and yet it hadn't. That the floor had not been smashed open, only that the metal under their feet had buckled up, right under where he was sitting, and that something slammed into them: no shrapnel, no bomb fragments in the cabin, nothing, but still his colleague was dead, torn apart, and all the others were able to walk away. A bomb and yet not a bomb. It didn't make sense.

On the operating table the orthopaedic surgeon stood still for a second or two as he looked down at what were possibly the worst injuries he had ever seen where there was still a recognisable leg. The skin was somehow still attached, although the muscles underneath were dead and mostly turned to mush. The bone was so badly fractured it was possible to concertina the limb from its full length up into a squashed flesh cube a quarter of the original size. If the bone had been whole, he could have saved the leg, patched up the soft tissue on the ward and then a slow rebuild of grafts and flaps. But the bone was gone, so there was nothing to build on and so the leg was amputated.

Strangest of all, he had seen it before: the bone at least. He'd seen it in four patients, none of whom got near a war zone except inside their own heads. They had all been 'jumpers' who had tried to kill themselves by jumping off a high building, jumpers rather than fallers because jumpers land on their feet and fallers twist and struggle in the air to escape their fate. Jumpers take all the impact of their fall on their feet and legs, and that was where he had seen bones concertina up into themselves like that. He'd done a fellowship in Baltimore, at the world's leading shock trauma unit – where the concept of the Golden Hour had been formulated – where the trauma unit was close by the psych building and where patients jumped off one roof (which wasn't high enough to kill) and (not directly) ended up in the operating theatre of the other.[3] He'd had two patients there, where their jump had ended with smashed heels, broken femurs and thighs, open fractures, shattered pelvises. They had ended up having trauma care and orthopaedic surgery at the same time, life and limb one and the same, just like he would do at Bastion. And he'd had a third and fourth patient when he returned to the UK – one off a 110-foot roof and one who'd jumped off an iron railway bridge: smashed heels, all the rest and damage to the lower spine. So all of them, like the Afghan patient who now lay on the operating table before him, with the same kinds of injuries: they had been hit very hard, very intense, very localised from below, with most of the impact going on their feet and legs. So it didn't matter where the hit came from, it had the same effect. Invisible energy, transmitted up limbs, destroying everything in its path. Do something about it. There was the problem he had come to find: the last of five patients, in the desert, destroyed by the heartbeat under the soil. Blast injury.

The orthopaedic surgeon began by writing a journal article that was read by others in the field who were also becoming interested, who were all coming at it from a slightly different angle, including someone who was taking time out from a medical degree to study bioengineering. And he introduced the orthopaedic surgeon to his supervisor. Bioengineering was exactly the right place for the orthopaedic surgeon to go because bioengineers also see the human body as a locomotor system. Bioengineering is where engineering solutions are brought to bear on medical conundrums, where a joint is seen as a hinge and a bone as a girder, and they can mathematise physical destruction. He found a home, then he found funding for it, and by the end of 2008, less than a year after the patient with the concertina-ed leg was brought to him at Bastion, the Blast Lab was born.[4]

It has a much grander name, and much better funding now: The Royal British Legion Centre for Blast Injury Studies (we call it 'CBIS'). But the questions it seeks to answer are the same as they were in 1915 when a military medic asked the scientists of Imperial: what are the effects of bomb wounds? What are the effects of blast injury? The answers, as they find out every day, are everywhere they look, however they go looking for them, from the twisted metal of the blasted vehicle flooring to the smallest micro-cell in the human body. Feature films that have huge explosions as part of their plot explain this really well. When the massive bomb has gone off, and the debris has settled and the hero has crawled out from wherever he or she has taken shelter, the first thing on the soundtrack is car alarms, hundreds of them, all going off at the same time, even if the car has no other visible damage apart from settling dust and a few scratches. It's the blast wave that does that, to a vehicle's electronics, invisibly, just like what it can do to all the human bodies in its impact zone. When you hear a car alarm set off by a blast on the news or in a film, you are hearing the alarm in the human body – damage, deep and long-lasting, already done.[5]

Blast injury was known and feared before 2008, but studying it was a matter of gathering statistics and working from them, whether hospital admission figures from Iraq or the early phase of Afghanistan, which came with increasingly desperate pleas to understand and brace for the new forms of casualty.[6]

Or data sets that turned up unexpectedly: such as a whole archive of material from the Zimbabwean War of Independence in the 1972–80 phase that described cheap and effective vehicle modifications to deflect the impact of blast from fields of Russian mines, whose siblings still litter Angola, Cambodia and Afghanistan.[7] But it was still only statistics: useful for building models and hypotheses, but limited.[8] To begin to answer the questions about blast injury, first it needed to be understood, and to be understood it needed to be simulated – recreate the injuries in an environment where they could be measured, quantified, studied. Slow them down, see what they do microsecond by microsecond, cell by cell, intervene.

Beyond copper walls and German shell samples available from the War Office, Imperial got equipment that could simulate the worst effects of blast on whatever material they chose. It consists of really big bits of kit, very heavy, very blasty (according to the medic who introduced the surgeon to the bioengineers in the first place), and initially they put them on the sixth floor of our building in South Kensington and no one entirely remembers how they got them up the stairs. But when the Lab became a Centre, everything was formalised and given a proper home, Level minus one on the lift buttons. Today meetings in Bioengineering are punctuated by distinct thuds coming from the basement labs under our offices. We don't tend to notice them any more, but we try to remember to explain them to visitors. The lead engineer, who works with the orthopaedic surgeon who started it all off, even has a personal tagline: 'I know how to hit things really hard and measure them.'[9] And they can talk to each other – engineers and medics in the same place. They can go next door and ask one another what is happening, and get an explanation, using whichever is most necessary, an equation or a CT scan.

One of the CBIS bioengineers was doing a public engagement with schoolchildren, who asked him if he had always wanted to work with explosives. He said he had, that if his eight-year-old self could see him when he started his job, he'd be really impressed that he could get paid to blow things up. And for a year or so, blowing things up, and filming them, slowing the film down so he could see every single thing that happened on the B of the Blast – at the very beginning – then measuring the physical effects, was enough. He was getting good hard data but also useful life lessons, such as that the novelty of blowing up a raw egg soon wore off. Egg bits went everywhere and were really difficult to clean up, and after a couple of days the shock lab equipment started to smell of rotten blasted-egg debris. So he stuck to tomatoes and oranges. And then something else happened that surprised him. He stopped being obsessed with blowing things up, and started being obsessed with protecting humans from what happens when things blow up.

He's the bioengineer who works on blast lung, and he has become every bit as preoccupied with breathing as MERT medics in their Chinooks. He wants to know why the architecture of lung tissue works the way it does, why long after the echo of the original blast has died away in the air it is still present in the lungs, still deadly, why lungs tear so easily and keep tearing. Lungs are the only tissue in humans to tear in this way (there's a biblical word for it, which is also the medical word – to be 'rent'). They are so very fine, and they are never at rest, and perhaps it has to do with fatigued areas, or local defects that are exacerbated by the blast wave and just go on and on collapsing. But in the meantime, until he has figured this out, blast lung is assumed in all patients close to an explosion, and treated immediately, and he is using his knowledge to design a material that can be added to body armour so that both the blast wave and the blast fragments can be resisted. He has colleagues who are working on the linings of heavy soldier boots so that a blast wave from below can be mitigated, and others who are making materials that can go on the floor of vehicles for the same purpose.[10]

It isn't just Imperial. There are sites all over the country and all over the world where research into the effects of the nightmare that is blast injury is ongoing, which all began at around the same time, 2008 or 2009, when the scourge of the IED began to be felt, urgently, bloodily. But the war in Afghanistan is now over, has been for several years, and history shows us how, beyond this initial emergency, this kind of progress can be stopped in its tracks, by factors more complicated to understand than war or blast – institutional resistance and inertia.

Take something that happens to 70 per cent of military amputees that causes them chronic pain and disrupts prosthetic use. It's becoming the most significant obstacle to a return to an active lifestyle, so they know a lot about it at Headley. This is heterotopic ossification (HO), where soft tissue that isn't bone turns to bone. Not bone growing oddly, but something that had never been a bone – like a nerve or a blood vessel or a muscle – ossifying, becoming a bone. Within months or years (HO is like that) it grows inside the amputation stump, following the line of whatever its original form was – long, winding spires following nerves, or webbing where it was blood vessels. It changes stump volumes completely and presses on other nerves and joints, causing pain, which is usually when a CT scan is ordered, and there it is, like coral: HO. It happens to civilians – just a few of them, who have hip replacements or spinal surgery, and it's relatively easy to treat, with medication and radiation. But it happens so often to military amputees that it is now officially classified as a wound-specific condition, and with complex casualty medication and radiation aren't always a match for ravaged inflammatory mechanisms and immune systems, so the only solution is more surgery. Sometimes the spire of HO can be removed on its own, but often it means more, higher amputation, an above-the-knee turning into a hemipelvectomy. No more chance of a prosthetic. Back in the chair, never out again.

There are several research projects into the causes and possible treatment of HO going on now, one of them at Imperial, and the consensus is that it's blast, complicated by genes and inflammation. For me as a historian the most important factor is that none of this is new. HO was identified a century ago, by a medical scientist working for the military in First World War France, who was handed over a ward full of soldier amputees whose stumps were persistently painful and couldn't take a prosthetic. The scientist used X-rays (one of the first to do so for medical research purposes) and found that there was bone where there shouldn't be bone. Then she looked at the records of their injury. All of the patients had received serious musculo-skeletal damage as a result of an exploding shell – blast injury – damage from the fragments and damage from the invisible wave of energy that passed through them at the same time. The blast wave, she concluded, was causing HO.[11] And then nothing. The scientist, Augusta Déjerine-Klumpke, died in 1927, and her work was lost. Not just her work, even the memory of her, despite her importance to medical history as a pioneering medical scientist who made significant contributions to the study of the structure and repair of human neuroanatomy. Then, in the twenty-first century, a whole new cohort of military amputee patients presented with persistent pain and difficulty with their prosthetics, and X-rays revealed bone growth where none should be, some of which can be removed surgically but not all. So they go on suffering while the scientists pick up threads laid down a century before and start to follow them again. Like with pain, what a terrible waste of time.

Not just military amputees. Nearly everyone who survived the 7/7 bombings in London and needed an amputation has developed the same thing: HO.[12] And I may be just a historian, but from where I sit the evidence looks persuasive that 70 per cent of anyone who loses a limb to a blast injury, be it bomb or mine or IED anywhere in the world, where the invisible wave passes through what's left of their body, that body will get the extra bone where bone should not be: HO. And pain and prosthetic malfunction will follow.

Everyone, in all the minefields or civil wars or battlegrounds, man, woman or child, will see some if not all of the complications of blast injury. I wrote this section on 22 March 2016, ten hours after the bombs in the airport and tube station in Brussels killed thirty-five and injured hundreds more. Many were in a railway carriage, just like in London, where the metal walls contain and concentrate the blast wave, magnifying its effects, meaning more energy absorbed by humans, blast lung and all the rest. Survivors were interviewed on television, covered in dust and minor lacerations, saying they were fine, even though they had been in the carriage where the bomb went off, and everyone who studies blast lung shouts at their television – 'Go to A&E, get a scan, you are not all right.' Five days later, another blast, in Lahore, killed seventy and injured almost three hundred. The Lahore blast was so large it could be heard several kilometres away, firing up car alarms all over that part of the city, just like in the films.

And then there's Afghanistan today, after the foreign armies have gone and taken Field Hospital Camp Bastion and all those other extraordinary medical facilities with them, leaving only ordinary ones behind. On 19 April 2016 a huge truck bomb went off in Kabul, obliterating an entire car park, its blast wave smashing every window for a wide radius, including those of the city's largest mosque. Kabul's ambulance service faced the very worst day since its founding in 2003. All fifteen of its vehicles were immediately rushed to the scene, removing victims to the city's hospitals. It looked like something from the Somme – some ambulances carried as many as twelve victims inside one vehicle, the seated packed in and over and around the stretchers. The doors of two vehicles broke off at the hinges because of the multiple heavy loads carried over eighty-three separate trips between the bomb site and the medical facilities.[13] It was the worst attack in the country's capital in fifteen years of war, remarkable even by Afghan standards. The next day it was reported that sixty-four people had been killed and 347 wounded, but that figure was likely to be on the low side for both categories.

All these survivors across the world will all get some variations of all the other things we are coming to understand at the cellular level at Imperial. Not just a known military cohort but an entire global population of blast casualty on every continent, living out the pain of the echo of the blast and its invisible armoury one difficult step and day at a time. For most of them there is no one watching, no one going back to the lab with what they've learned to try to make it better. So what happens at places like Imperial can only ever be a start.

24

Mark Ormrod (6)

The way I look after my prosthetic limbs is the same
as the way I used to look after my rifle.[1]

Mark Ormrod, blog post, 2015

RESEARCH HAPPENS in places other than Imperial. Other universities, hospitals, government laboratories and sometimes, exceptionally (because this is Mark Ormrod), in private houses and private lives. Mark Ormrod works every day at finding the best way to live as he is now. He may not be inside a science facility, but he is his own experiment, testing his limits and consolidating his gains, even when they are small and not what he was hoping for. He's making YouTube videos now, and in one of them he dances a bit before beginning his workout. Pretty good dancing, shoulders and hips working in rhythm – he's come on a long way since learning to stand at Headley, learning to dance upright for his wedding. He's grateful every Christmas Eve, the anniversary of the day of his wounding (and he celebrates by throwing some weights around at a gym session), the day he didn't die, but mainly that he gets to go and have Christmas Day with the girl who sat by his side on the floor, and his three children, but he's also grateful for the people that help him with the ongoing research project that is life as Mark Ormrod.

Mark left the military in 2010, but he still runs his life as if he was a Marine. They made him efficient, resourceful, a planner. But it was only after he was injured that he learned just how much these skills would mean in his new life. Each of his three prosthetics, which he got from the Hanger Prosthetics and Orthotics company, cost a great deal more than his rifle, and he inspects them and maintains them as carefully as the weapon that guarded his life. There's no sergeant-major looking over his shoulder, but then no sergeant-major has ever been as critical of Mark as he is of himself now (occasionally, and at their peril, he takes private clients as a personal trainer and coach). Each day he moves forward, and at the end of each day he prepares for the next.[2] He makes a list, every night, of what he wants out of the next day, on a piece of paper or on his phone. He puts them in order of importance, sets a deadline, and then it's the first thing he sees when he wakes up after a proper amount of the deepest sleep he can get.

Mark has thought a lot about goals since those that were set in his first meeting at Headley with the team that is going to get their patients back up on to their new feet. He knows that, without goals, someone in a tight spot withers and succumbs to their circumstances early.[3] He's seen those people leave Headley no matter what, in a wheelchair. But not him:

> Have you seen that person who faces the same set of circumstances but sets themselves goals and has focus and direction? What happens to them? They thrive!
>
> Once you have goals it awakens a drive inside you and makes you feel alive and like you have massive purpose […] if you aim at nothing, you'll hit nothing […] [Goals] will challenge you, excite you and make you feel alive, the way you're supposed to feel.

And just in case things change (as if they'd dare), he always has a crash bag packed, like they do in the army: small, carry-on size, full of the things that are essential to him, for his prosthetics, which he can't afford to forget, because if he ever did, he wouldn't be able to walk.

Every evening, his crash bag stowed away and his list made, he prepares his clothes for the next day. He changes a lot, and changing clothes as an amputee is complicated and takes longer than otherwise, so he lays out what he needs, in order. He looks at his list and sees what prosthetics he'll need. Gym prosthetics usually, because he works out most days, and then different legs for walking and stairs. A set of work clothes, trousers and shoes, and if he has a function in the evening, a smart suit. Clothes are always tricky for an amputee. They don't fit properly on their new body shape – worst of all on a double above-knee amputation. Mark has a 32-inch waist but needs to buy a size 34 so that the shorts (because, like most amputees, he wears shorts with almost everything) are big enough to fit over his sockets without being too tight, and look smart. Same problem at the gym, which is where he does most of his work: the fit isn't right and gets in the way. So Mark goes custom, even for the gym, and has his gear specially made for him by a tailor on Jermyn Street in London. The tailor has been going to Headley for a while now, because she understands that severe casualty poses practical problems on top of the physical complications, so she custom-makes shirts and jackets that fit over sockets and stoma bags, with trousers in all kinds of leg length, and she even brings walking sticks that do the job of crutches but which look considerably more dapper (hand-carved ebony woods with buffalo horn handle and engraved initials).

Mark keeps his office tidy, paperwork to a minimum, stacked up tidily at night ready for him in the morning, and he keeps his inbox and his phone stripped back of anything that isn't necessary. He backs up computer devices regularly, as we're all supposed to. His car is vital to him. He drives one-handed, and he really can't do anything else, like reach for a ringing phone or a bag slipping off a seat, so everything needs to be exactly as he wants it before he sets out, all complications anticipated. Complications might mean dependency. Mark has been dependent, while he was brought out of the desert, while he lay in the back of a Chinook, while he sweated through fevers at Birmingham and pain at Headley, and he doesn't care for it. Dependency is chaos, being overwhelmed. Preparation beats it all back.

Life as an amputee is complicated and tiring, even for Mark, who is young and energised. Life as an amputee requires him to be an athlete, every day, even though he isn't aiming for an Olympics of any kind. It took him a while to realise this, and when he accepted that from now on he was going to have to be an athlete as well as an amputee, it gave him structure and order. He's clear in his own mind what his life means, and he's good at explaining exactly what that means, every day:

> Being a double above-knee amputee [...] takes between 300 and 500 per cent more energy to do anything than it would for a normal able-bodied person. If you woke up in the morning and spent the entire day jogging around from one place to the next instead of walking, if while you stood still you were jogging on the spot, and if you wore a weighted vest when you were doing things like getting up off the floor or standing up from a chair, that's pretty much the same level of energy that it takes for me to get through a normal day as a full-time prosthetic user.

Wherever you look in Mark's home, things are ready for him so he can go on being exactly who he needs to be, that day and the next. He thinks about everything, every single thing, that he eats. He always has breakfast, no skipping. And healthy snacks, ready prepared, the preparation thing in everything. He drinks plenty of water, starts the day with hot water and maybe a slice of lemon because it gets his digestion going. He does all this because, like the prosthetists at Headley, he knows that weight fluctuations are complications that it's better to avoid. Soldiers, especially those who serve on the front line, can eat anything they like, because their metabolism simply burns off excess and they come back from there thin and undernourished, a real problem in Critical Care at Bastion or

Birmingham. So by the time they get to Headley they can't eat what they like but they do, and usually this means putting on weight. It took Mark about a year to put on muscle mass but take off weight, and he did it by cutting out junk food, carbohydrates and alcohol. Instead he kept his body energised with smaller regular meals, which helped but weren't enough for the demands he made on his body, especially once he went back in the gym almost full-time, at Headley and then back home. He's still working on what constitutes the perfect diet for him.

Back and forth, a bit like Headley, gym work, results, mobility and looking good, as good as he has ever looked, and then exhaustion, falling, failure. Start again, new routine, fail but maybe fail better. This kind of original research is always difficult, never straightforward, and Mark doesn't have a supervisor to guide him. He's supervisor, researcher and student all in one. The 300–500 per cent energy demands aren't just about the gym; they are about every waking moment of every day. The only time he didn't need the extra energy was when he was sleeping, in his bedroom, the one with the crash bag ready in the corner and the next day's clothes hanging on the wardrobe door. Otherwise, every step, every lift up from a chair and every single stair – more energy, and still more – not just the increasingly technical exercise regimes he devised for himself in the gym. Mark's is a body never really at rest. To get it to function as he wanted, he once again had to choose who to listen to, and finally he chose to listen to what his new body was trying to tell him. Not standard academic language but clear:

> There's not much point having a killer body that looks good if you're constantly miserable trying to maintain it and every day feels like a struggle, believe me when I say that because I've been through that process several times myself.

Every day feels like a struggle. A struggle, as he puts it, while wearing a weighted vest. Mark has a family, and he knows the impact of his research project on them. His family see him when he struggles, when he flings aside whatever he has been working on because, no matter what he does, no matter the pain, nothing is working. He knows, above all, that a lot of the time the focus of the family is on him, and how he's doing, and that just acknowledging that is helpful. Also they have what he calls 'Fat Boy Fridays', when the entire family gets to eat what they want (ice cream mostly, judging from his Twitter feed pictures), not just what is working for Mark that particular month. When his children run and fall, Mark can go to them himself, and help them up (by carefully engaging the right muscles in his whole body and all his strength). So he's become the dad he thought he should be, not dependent, but still something of a challenge for his children, starting with the eldest, his daughter.

Other children, at school or locally, would ask why her dad had funny legs and a hook instead of a hand. At first he tried to spare her the sight of him in front of her friends and stopped picking her up at school. He considered never going to the school ever again, so they would forget and she wouldn't be the girl with that dad. Ultimately he let his daughter choose who to listen to, and she told him she could take it and that she wanted it to be him who stood at the school gates and waved her in and came back at the end of the day to collect her. The children who saw him were curious and they asked her lots of questions, questions that were complicated for her to answer, and it got her down.

Together they came up with something that might help. Mark had started doing motivational speaking by this point, so he had some practice in explaining himself to audiences. They decided he would speak at her school assembly. He thought it couldn't possibly be harder than a room full of top execs in suits. But it was. Mark was more nervous than he had been for a long time: rows of little faces looking up at him, one of them his girl, and he didn't want to let her down. But he didn't, and he took all their questions and explained everything, and then there were no more questions, or if they were, someone who had been paying attention in his assembly explained the answer to the others. He has more children now, and he expects to do more assemblies because 'I don't want to cause any problems for them going through school as I know it can be tough enough anyway without anything extra to deal with.' He's prepared now: speech for assembly, crash bag in the corner, next day's clothes on a hanger, family behind and in front of him.

25

Sockets and Stumps and Science

A PROSTHETIC MEANS 'an artificial part supplied to remedy a deficiency'. But always artificial, and not, in the words of the design historian, with much chance of ever matching the performance of the real thing. The problem is the stump-and-socket model, the impermanence, the changeability, the inefficiency of the interface, the pain. One solution seems to be to take changeability out of the equation by replacing the limb permanently.

There are two models of permanent limb replacement. The first is transplantation: where a donated limb is surgically attached to a stump. This is already happening with hands and arms. The surgery is straightforward – no techniques that aren't already in use – but nothing else about the procedure is. Prior to surgery the immune system is suppressed, and suppressed hard, and then it is suppressed by heavy medication loads for as long as the transplant remains attached. There's no forgetting it's a transplant for the patient, because they have to look for signs of rejection every day, painstakingly. Rejection starts as a rash or a change in skin tone and can appear anywhere on the new limb. In the early stages it doesn't hurt, but every little thing has to be reported to the transplant surgeon. Limb transplant can only be done if the patient can manage the heavy immune-suppressant regime (and not everyone can).

Transplants are not just about soft tissue and bone. They

also reconnect nerves to brain, and although it takes a while, some sensation does eventually return as the nerves and brain rewire themselves. This process seems to be about length, so the longer the limb being transplanted, the longer it will take to register sensation. Sensation is needed not just so the person can touch and feel again, but also so that their own body can protect them – so pain can be registered. Ideally this means the restoration of nociceptor pain, the really useful form of pain that tells the brain that damage and danger are imminent and to react. With hand and arm transplants some function can be returned (but it takes intensive, specialist rehab) to the point at which patients can write, feed and clean themselves, and when they speak, their hands have begun to be expressive again, vague but discernible motions of body language. None of this works for legs. Return of sensation isn't really relevant; limb transplants aren't load-bearing – they can't take weight – so there is no possibility of ever leaving the wheelchair behind.

So if we are a very long way from leg transplants, what are the other options? Something permanently attached, that gets away from the stump-and-socket model but which can take weight and doesn't need the sledgehammer immune-suppressant regime. There is another technique called osseo-integration, where metal prosthetics are attached directly and permanently on to the bones in the stump. It's an integration technique because the idea is that the metal prosthetic will integrate with the bone to create a whole – a new join, not something detachable or changeable. No more socket: just a stump with a metal clip for a prosthetic sticking out of the end.

As with limb transplants, none of the components of osseo-integration is new, just the way they are being used. We know that bones can grow new pieces of themselves, which is how fractures heal if they are set right. We also know that bone cells will regrow on a surface not made of bone and that the result-ant integrated area can take weight and generate movement. Osseo-integration is what makes knee and hip and dental implants work, and the vertebral screws that pin together smashed bones. So osseo-integration at amputation stumps builds on all these things that we know already work.

Unlike limb transplantation, osseo-integration is being done on amputees today. The surgery involves attaching a bespoke metal implant, measured to match the existing or former limb, to a neatly trimmed bone end. This is the thing that will replace the socket. This implant is designed to be transcutaneous, which means that the other end of the implant sticks out of the stump, so a plastic surgeon has to close up the soft tissue of the stump carefully around the sides of the implant end. There is a coupling at the end of the implant to which prosthetics can then be attached. The coupling is designed to break, like a ski binding, if it comes under pressure.

After surgery the patient goes back to rehab, where they and their new implant learn how to take loads again. Specialist physios help them develop the bone density, millimetre by millimetre, so that eventually they will be able to put their weight down on their new legs through their new implant. Bone grows and becomes denser at the interface as its owner moves and places loads on it – just as runners have better bone density than people who don't move around so much. Loads equal density equals a good level of osseo-integration. The first time patients put weight on their big legs at Headley it's all about balance. With osseo-integration it's about load and developing bone density – growing something back that had been taken away. That's where this system has it over the stump-and-socket replacement model. Soft tissue, like skin and muscles worked over bone remnants, isn't supposed to take load and responds inefficiently when it has to. Bone ends in stumps don't increase their density, because the bone has nothing to engage or interface with. Implants promote regrowth – not much, but significant.

Integrated implants mean that prosthetics are attached to the skeleton again, not a socket which is controlled by muscles that weren't ever supposed to do that. The patient's brain says Leg Lift and Go Upstairs, and it does. The prosthetic leg clips on to the implant in twenty seconds, without the palaver of socks and linings and stumps being manoeuvred into sockets. Integrated implants work well for amputees with knees. Above the knee, and things are not so clear. Above the knee osseo-integrated implants remind us that this is a very new technique and one where we do not yet know the long-term outcomes, because there haven't yet been any long-term outcomes to know. No one has had one of these for more than five years. We know a few things: that patients can't run with integrated implants, that the implants can still break and that managing tissue around the bit of implant that sticks out through the skin is difficult. Apart from our gums and nail beds, human skin is designed to be a closed system, with no direct access for micro-organisms. If the transcutaneous section of the implant gets infected, it can spread, and ultimately the whole system can fail. Very few of the patients who end up back in their chairs back in their surgeons' consulting rooms are suitable candidates for osseo-integration. But that doesn't change the fact that sockets are the worst of their problems every day of the week, every week of the year. If someone tells an amputee there's a system where the socket can be replaced, they don't hear anything else after that.

So another way is to make the socket better. Make it smarter. Make it tell the patient when things are starting to go wrong: temperature, moisture, weight slowly shifting to the wrong place, red marks that last for longer than ten minutes, muscle strain, deep tissue damage, ulcers. Or just simple things, like they aren't walking quite as well or efficiently as they might. Too much energy being expended for not enough effort. Choose who you listen to, and one day they will be able to listen to their socket because it's going to ring them on their phone and tell them how it's feeling. Optimum stump health – there's an app for that.

How to make a socket smart? Take existing sensor technology and the idea of wearables and put them together – sensors inside a socket. One model currently being researched is a paper-thin liner that goes inside the socket to take measurements. Hold out your hand, fingers spread, and then take your other hand and make a fist. Put it in the palm of your flat hand and then wrap your fingers around your fist. As you move your fist about, your fingertips sense every muscle and tendon as it works. The smart socket is the same principle. It's shaped like a cobweb made of flat, plasticised film, with a suite of sensors on every point. It fits down inside the socket, between the exterior and the elastic sock lining that goes over the stump.

When the stump is inserted in the socket and the patient stands up and moves, the sensors transmit data via Bluetooth to processors stuck on the back of the outside of the socket casing. There's lots of spare room all over the leg and the technology is light, so no extra weight.[1] If everything works well (and the batteries for transmitters charge properly, which is the main problem at the moment), this gives sockets the potential to be their own little data-processing centres. And the sensor data that spins out from their web is pure gold, almost infinitely useful.

Most importantly of all, and whatever the eventual model will be, smart sockets tell their wearer when something is going wrong: too hot, wrong loading, sweat, swelling, deep tissue dysfunction, balance wrong, symmetry off. It's an early warning system, so adjustments can be made quickly – sit down, but only for a few minutes, use a wipe to clean an overheated, sweaty stump, fix the padding, get out in front of the problem and shut it down. Nearly as important as telling the wearer what is wrong, the smart socket also tells when things are going right. Balance, weight loading, symmetry, gait. Press a button and the wearer and their physio can see a graph that plots their progress now against progress they made last month, so they can see the accumulation of things going right, and keep doing them.

The really smart thing about the idea of a smart socket is that it gives everyone involved in the injury a shared language, for things that go wrong and for things that go right. Smart socket data could be used by prosthetists, physios or Paralympic coaches for repairs, maintenance, improvements, refinements. Shared languages, as the pain consultant will testify, are essential. It takes the guesswork out if the patient can watch their own biofeedback in real time, with their physio, seeing what effect new exercises or step patterns have, right there on a screen. A shared language means that whenever they get a new physio or move to a new NHS catchment area, they hand over a data stick, and they never quite have to start from scratch. A smart socket makes a smarter patient – expert in their own condition, with stats to prove it. This is where Mark Ormrod's personal research programme and the technical wizardry of university research departments meet.

This could be a significant step forward, if it works out as it should. Smart sockets will suit the global amputee population because, although they may not have 3D printers (currently the solution to everything, if you believe the gospel according to TED), they do have smartphones. Smart socket sensor arrays, whatever their model, will be small. Fit the sensor in the socket, clip on the hardwear, download the app and off it goes. Upload the data and study it, upload the data to the Cloud, contribute to a new kind of global analytics. What works all over the world, for everyone taking the same journey on whatever kind of road is laid out before them. A new meaning for the global amputee population, becoming part of their own solution. Hurry up, I say to the quietly brilliant PhD student whose work this is, whose hands shake because we are all watching him when he puts the batteries in Dave Henson's processor on the day he first tests it at the running track at Battersea Park. Hurry up, not just because it's a cold day and it's getting dark, but because this is so important.

If we can have a smarter socket, how about a smarter stump? This is what Dave Henson is working on, now he is back from Rio. He wants to build on the initial insights from back before he was injured, when physios and surgeons in the UK told surgeons at Bastion that the through-knee amputation was the best, leaving as much leg to work with as possible. His through-knee stump is evidence of that. He has a complete femur kneecap and an entire calf muscle that a plastic surgeon at Bastion carefully connected up to some surviving tendons, bundled up and tucked into the soft tissue around Dave's remaining bone, just in case. This is all material that could be usefully recycled into some kind of knee – and any kind of knee is better than no knee at all. So, using maths, and scans and the kind of engineering models that are second nature to him, Dave is finding ways to optimise the surgical anatomy of the stump. He is aiming to give surgeons a formal anatomical model to guide them when they are presented with a leg blasted into fragments, random avulsive injuries, seemingly chaotic. They will be able to compare their patient with the Henson model and handle bones, muscles, tendons, ligaments on the operating table in a way that later on will be useful to the patient and their physio and their prosthetist. They will make their decisions about all the elements in the stump they are about to create, not just in case or just for now or for the time in the prosthetic workshop, but for a whole lifetime. The Henson model will take into account likely gait patterns, functionality, pain. It will project how the new stump will affect bone density in areas, such as hips, that will have to take more strain than they were originally intended for, so how to avoid creating areas that are likely to develop osteoarthritis and other conditions that cause fractures. The model won't just be for surgeons; it will also guide engineers and designers in the development of better technology. That's what optimised stump surgical anatomy is; if there has to be a stump, then make it the best possible, most useful, least painful stump there can be.

There are other ways to make the stump be all it can be. Make the skin on the stump better, more resilient, able to take the loads thumping down on it with every step. We do already have this kind of skin, on the palms of our hands but mainly on the heels of our feet. Here it is ten times thicker than anywhere else on the body, and it's compliant, not brittle, it doesn't break under strain of the big heel bone (the calcaneus) in the base of your foot thumping down on it with every step you take. When your shoes don't fit properly, you get blisters on your ankle bones, on your toes, everywhere else, but not your heel, because here the skin has adapted to take the pressure.[2] There's a gene (HOXA13, if you're interested) that determines protein levels in the epidermis, and that's what makes your heels tough as old boots. If there could be heel skin on a stump where the residual bone comes thumping down with every step, then all those problems that come from ordinary skin not being great under strain might be resolved.[3]

It would mean reprogramming the skin at the genetic level, but this is another thing we already do for something else (hair transplants: move a hair follicle and it goes on making hair wherever it gets put because the skin around it changes into becoming hair-follicle-supporting skin). So cells that know they are heel skin cells could be transplanted into skin on other parts of the body (provided that body has heels left), which then start to operate like a heel and start to toughen up. We are only just starting to do this in the lab, but when it's ready, one day, HOXA13 can go in a cream, and the amputee can use their smart socket data to see exactly where they should put it on their stump. All of this research is at an early stage; when I wrote this, the scientists who came up with it were just starting to fill out the forms for funding. That's how science works. Someone has a really, really smart idea that could change the world, and then they fill out forms for funding.

*

Postscript
Both projects got funding.

26

Complex Outcomes, Chronic Pain and PTSD

Pain is SO complicated. *(historian to pain consultant)*
No shit, Emily. *(pain consultant to historian)*[1]

FOR MOST OF THE UNEXPECTED CASUALTY COHORT, the pain begun at the point of wounding is still going on. It is still too early to say if this will be a problem in the long term (because we aren't in the long term yet), but all the indications are that it will be, because, beyond the military context, pain is still extremely challenging to treat. We don't yet have (as the medical textbooks say) a theory of pain that allows a structured approach to its mitigation. True analgesia – achieving an absence of pain in a waking human life – is a long way off.

The pain consultant who put together the system that worked from Afghanistan through Birmingham and beyond Headley is all too aware that his work is unfinished. He has always seen pain and its treatment as a continuum, so he would ideally like to see the Military Pain Team evolve into something else that can offer their patients much longer-term care: something that can involve 'the thirty-year, 13,000-mile pain service'. At the moment he can't do that. Once his military patients are discharged, they move into the NHS, who currently manage their conditions, including pain. That's another story, and one that isn't yet written or ready to be written, because although the results of this transition are mixed, recently some ex-military patients have been able to re-access some military medical facilities, which is good for them and helpful to the NHS. It isn't yet a formal, clarified relationship, but people are working really hard to get this done, to incorporate the military and the NHS into one system of care for complex casualty. But the ends of wars are tricky places to makes plans in (see the various history sections in this book), and we aren't there yet.

Although the NHS pain service may operate differently from the military, the understandings of pain are aligned (although not their language – one disadvantage of moving out of the military pain service is that patients leave behind the pain ladder, with its three or four clear steps up and down). So for everyone, from the point of wounding, and through definitive reconstruction and treatment, any pain experienced by the patient is termed 'acute'. If pain is still hanging around after six months and the underlying cause of pain has been treated and accounted for, pain is said to have become 'chronic'. In military casualty, even if the underlying cause of pain can never be fully treated and accounted for, it's the same thing. Chronic pain is treated as a condition in its own right, in addition to or beyond the original injury. The relationship between the nerves and brain is no longer straightforward. Damage and danger may have passed (even if temporarily), yet the pain outlasts them, for no particular purpose. Chronic pain has become a fact of life.

The treatment for chronic pain is not standard, apart from everyone agreeing that it needs a 'multi-disciplinary approach and should involve more than one therapeutic modality'.[2] So research into chronic pain relief goes the same way as treatment – a maze of complex, complicated strands looking at drug dosage strengths, drug dose combinations, nerve blocks, hypnosis, acupuncture, steroid injections, oral therapies (tablets), topical therapies (creams). There was even a study that looked at swearing as a response to pain. When you experience pain, if you swear (official scientific term: pain-related catastrophising), then the sensation of pain is somewhat lessened. It was a serious study, but probably not much use for soldiers because it only works with people who don't swear much to start with, and the analgesic affects are short-term.[3]

And in the midst of this, something quietly new, a possibility that resonates particularly with the pain consultant who told me about it while I was trying to make sense of the maze that is chronic pain research. Chronic pain was the reason he tried to prevent pain as early as possible, from the point of wounding. He did this, not as part of a research project, but because his entire professional life had taught him that chronic pain is about a nervous system that knows it has been hurt before, and is extremely sensitive to being hurt again. Chronic pain is remembered pain. Chronic pain is the brain remembering much too well how to react to pain. Memory is a strong force in humans and an equally strong force in their pain. The damage and the danger may have passed, but the cry of pain in the body, where the body seeks to protect itself, is left behind. It isn't the same cry of pain that happened at the point of wounding. It has been intensified by time, and its activation is rewired beyond logic or biology, so the memory of pain, and therefore pain, can be triggered by things that are normally innocuous – or by anything at all, any sensory input or change in circumstance. It's no way for a brain to be. Or a nervous system – this extreme sensitivity happens all along the pain network, from nerves to brain. So the entire system has lost the ability to discriminate between damage and ordinary, non-harmful stimuli.

So chronic pain is not about inputs but about a new state of the brain.[4] And this new state is complex, dynamic. As the scientists working on it say, in both a technically precise and unexpectedly poetic finding: 'the essence of central sensitisation is a constantly changing mosaic of alterations in membrane excitability.' This state, say the scientists (less poetically), represents a major target for therapeutic intervention. The pain consultant thinks this will mean not only drugs to calm the excitability but also the development of therapies – the kind he has advocated, asking, talking, understanding – that enable the patient and their brain and its membranes to calm down, permanently. Whatever the intervention, at its heart will be unpicking the memory of pain, stitch by stitch, until the conscious mind has helped the brain find its normal response levels again.[5]

*

Chronic pain is pain remembered. Because of an acute insult, the brain rewires itself so it no longer reacts normally to stimuli. This abnormality goes on long after the insult is over, because the brain doesn't have the ability to change back on its own. This explanation works equally well for post-traumatic stress disorder. PTSD is stress remembered. Because of an acute incident the brain rewires itself so that it no longer reacts normally. Long after the incident is past, the abnormality goes on because the brain doesn't have the ability to change back. Dr Bessel van der Kolk, medical director of the world's leading PTSD research and treatment centre (the Trauma Centre at the Justice Resource Institute in Brookline, Massachusetts), who wrote the first integrative text on the effects of psychological trauma, puts it in proper scientific terms:

> Long after a traumatic experience is over it may be reactivated at the slightest hint of danger and mobilize disturbed brain circuits and secrete massive amounts of stress hormones. This precipitates unpleasant emotions, intense physical sensations and impulsive and aggressive actions.[6]

We are still not yet able, as with so much else, to assess the long-term psychological effect of deployment in Afghanistan on British service personnel. There is a consensus that around one in twenty-five service personnel will experience PTSD in some form as a result of military service, which is about the same level of mental disorder that is expected in non-military populations. That's about all the consensus on offer at the moment. Some of those engaging with the problem from a military point of view think it is a massive understatement, and others think it is dramatically overstating it. I think it has been wrongly stated. I think that there is a real lack of diagnostic clarity on anything to do with the brain after trauma, and we need that before we can agree numbers. I also think that the unexpected survivors of blast injury will be a key component in our ability to achieve clarity, because our investigations of the complexity of their casualty are already generating new, more precise diagnostic forms. These will be of service whether the point of wounding is physical or psychological.

Think back to the altered brain state of chronic pain and PTSD. It is important to think of them together for two reasons. First reason: where they occur together, each makes the other one so much worse (medical term: 'co-morbidity') and, separately, much more difficult to treat. At Headley physios understood the effect of pain on every other aspect of their patients' lives. By the time their patients become veterans, this has largely been forgotten. Mostly, chronic pain and PTSD are treated separately. Second reason: we should think of PTSD and chronic pain together because the latest research on both subjects clearly indicates that similar treatment models work in both cases.

This is not news. Thirteen years ago a study for the American Department of Veterans Affairs was really clear about the co-morbidity and its outcomes. Chronic pain and PTSD 'co-occur at a high rate and may interact in such a way as to negatively impact the course of either disorder'.[7] It's not really very surprising. A flash of pain or other random stimulus reminds the sufferer of the traumatic event. Sufferers become anxious and depressed as a result of their sensitivity, and the physiological response to the memory of trauma increases blood flow, which probably increases pain sensations. And round and round they go, gradually losing control of their lives. The authors of the study noted that there had been no 'studies investigating the efficacy of tailoring treatments for individuals for which pain and PTSD co-occur', and that this was unfortunate because 'such studies could significantly advance theory development and improve treatment efficacy'. They concluded:

> Overall it would be important to help patients with both pain and PTSD to understand the ways that these two disorders may maintain each other [then] their high levels of distress and disability may possibly decrease and they will be able to obtain a more positive quality of life.

We are, I think, finally in a place where the understanding of chronic pain and the understanding of PTSD are aligned. Repairing the effects of PTSD and chronic pain is about restoring the state of the brain to what it was before the point of wounding. We aren't yet in a place where treatment modes are aligned, but we are getting there. Medication can help bring calmness, sleep, but it is only a step on the way. Restoring the brain to normal response levels requires not just the understanding of scientists and therapists but also the understanding of patients. Good therapy in both cases is about paying attention to physical sensations – to the random stimuli that shouldn't set off reactions normally – recognising them and labelling them and seeing how they change when the pain or the PTSD spikes in their brain. Then, when everyone knows what they are, they can begin to work on them.

*

Ten years after the publication of the article on the co-morbidity of chronic pain and PTSD, our understanding has moved on. Researchers now talk about a 'co-morbidity cluster' because there is a third element to be considered in the diagnosis or mis-diagnosis of PTSD. It's the other acronym we all know from modern warfare: TBI – traumatic brain injury.[8] TBI is injury to the brain caused by trauma to the head, by a hit or a knock, or a bullet or a fragment. Sometimes the injury causes concussion, but not always. We know about it from sports injury, but TBI also accounts for one in four of all military casualties. TBI can cause everything from coma and severe disability to migraines and dizziness. It also causes depression, nightmares, insomnia and suicidal thoughts, which is why, months after the injuries themselves are thought to have physically healed, TBI is often misdiagnosed as PTSD.

Remember Robert Lawrence, on his way home from Tumbledown Mountain in 1982. Pain at the point of wounding after the high-velocity rifle shot and its shock wave tore out 45 per cent of his brain, pain for hours after, for hours during surgery, untreated post-operative pain, excruciating pain during his brain scan, pain in the aircraft that bought him home. A quarter of a century of crippling pain since then.[9] In an interview in 2007 he spoke angrily of the consequences of his injury, which have altered his behaviour and personality, and he did so primarily in the language of his PTSD diagnosis, saying that the worst injuries were to his mind.

Today it is clear that none of his injuries should be seen separately from the others. The researchers in 2011 are very clear that chronic pain, PTSD and TBI are always linked and that 'it is essential that […] studies recognise the close association between these areas of morbidity as markers of common pathophysiology, inter-related outcomes and therapy targets.' In other words, they shouldn't be seen or treated separately. No one should hive off psychological problems and ignore the big dent in the patient's head, the one he got from the high-velocity rifle bullet or the piece of IED. There is, in the quietly damning words of researchers, 'an entirely artificial dichotomy between neurological and psychiatric morbidity in TBI as a whole and military TBI in particular'.[10]

This brings us back to blast injury. On 9 June 2016, the

week before I wrote this paragraph, research findings were published that go a long way to clarifying the brain's reaction to trauma – specifically, blast trauma. From eight human cases the study found evidence that blast injury caused damage to the brain that lasted for years and was easily mistaken for PTSD. Not just evidence but a specific physical phenomenon that doesn't even have an acronym yet, although I hope it gets one because the brand-new technical term for it, 'interface astroglial scarring', is unlikely to catch on.

I say eight 'cases', because these were not patients. They were brain samples from eight US service personnel who had experienced blast in Iraq or Afghanistan and who had subsequently died. Three of the eight had died directly as a result of their exposure to an IED within days or weeks of their casualty, usually through a variety of brain haemorrhages. The other five had taken much longer to die after their exposure to the blast wave – from seven months to many years – and their causes of death ranged from suicide by gunshot wound to a variety of drug overdoses. None of their death certificates referred to head injuries. Instead they were all listed as having suffered with the classic PTSD symptoms: headaches, anxiety, depression, insomnia, chronic, unrelievable pain. All of them had been diagnosed with and treated for PTSD. And all of them had brain tissue samples banked at various locations in the United States.

When the scientists put those brain tissue samples under a microscope, they found they all had one thing in common: scarring to particular cells in the brain. Astroglia cells aren't the glamour cells of the brain carrying all the information around. They are more like scaffolding or tiling in the brain, providing the structural and chemical support to the neuronal cells (which do carry all the information around). In all eight cases astroglia cells, in areas of the brain where white (communications) and grey matter (processing) interface, showed exactly the same signs of scarring. Hence the name, interface astroglial scarring.[11] Scarring, wherever it occurs, indicates that tissue has been damaged to the extent that its internal physical architecture has been changed. Scarring fades when healing has been completed, so its continued presence indicates an incomplete process of recovery or permanent damage. Astro-glial scarring can occur as a result of other conditions (such as stroke or concussion or infection), and it isn't always a bad thing – glial scarring protects the more delicate, vital neuronal cell structures and therefore brain function. But the kind of astroglial scarring on the blast injury samples was different and indicated an entirely different level of severity – tissue damage that was both substantial and non-reversible.

Not just non-reversible. The scientists observed smaller amounts of scarring in those who had died soon after the blast, and 'prominent' or 'severe' scarring in those who had taken longer to go.[12] The scarring – the tissue damage – had grown and worsened with time. And the scientists only found this extreme form of scarring in cases where the patient had been exposed to a blast wave. Blast caused the original injury and then went on making it worse, for years. No such scars existed on patients with normal head injury, brain damage or con-cussion, and none on the control study of uninjured brains. Scarring, on the brains of the blasted, clear as day on a slide under a microscope, eight times, blasted forward, imprinted on the infrastructure of the human brain. The scars look like fine brown dust. More dust and fines, from the war in the desert to death in another desert at home, just as bleak.[13]

One of the scientists who undertook the study has a strong sense of history (what better kind of scientist can there be?), and he wants to look at brain tissue samples from shell shock casualties from the First World War to see if he can find the same scar dust there, because:

> Scientific literature from the past 100 years shows that a substantial percentage of blast-exposed service members have persistent neurological or behavioural symptomol-ogy [...]

Our findings suggest that for the first time, there might be a predictable pattern of physical damage to the human brain after blast exposure, which standard clinical neuroimaging techniques currently cannot detect [...]

We anticipate reconsideration about pathophysiology underlying the neuropsychiatric sequelae that follow blast exposure and also innovative approaches to diagnosis and treatment.[14]

*

This is an early stage – when scientists talk about 'anticipating reconsideration', this is technical language for 'there is a long way to go'. What it also means is that blast injury research, as a specialised topic and driven by the cohort of unexpected survivors, has produced a finding that could transform the way we diagnose PTSD. It gives us the means to be clear about the presence of persistent, worsening physical damage to the brains of sufferers. What it doesn't give us, yet, is an indication of how we treat that damage, make the scarring go away, restore the brain to normal function. Understanding the condition will help. But understanding won't be treatment, as it is in cases of PTSD and chronic pain for which there is no longer any sign of physical damage. But at least everyone will know where they stand.

*

It is all part of my answer to the hard questions asked by the unexpected survivor cohort about what has happened to them and what is going to happen to them, and all the others like them all over the world. The answer is hard – that's what makes this such a heavy reckoning. The deal for their lives was a difficult one because extreme resuscitation makes extreme demands on its survivors – not just those surviving blast injury, but mostly. Every day we are coming to understand just how difficult, because the effects of blast injury are complex and persistent and worsening. Every physiological system that makes us human is affected by blast, from our inflammatory mechanism to our brain structure. We don't yet have clinical solutions for many of these problems, but we are, in the meantime, trying to find them. It is the existence of the cohort that has enabled us to understand all of this, to provide a model for investigations into really complicated human casualty that we do not yet quite understand. Because of the cohort we know how to start looking for the terms of deals we have yet to do. We will be doing them, because we live in a world that increasingly demands from its medics what they demanded of themselves back during the small war fought far away – that they use all the means and skills at their disposal to refuse to let us die.

Epilogue

Medics

After each patient who died I got this feeling [...]
I think we all got it. I expect we all got it.

Paul Roach, *Citizen Surgeon*

AFTER SERVING AT THE SOMME from the first day (1 July 1916)
until the last (19 November 1916) without so much as a scratch,
a stretcher-bearer finally made it home to London for some
leave. For a day he greeted his family and saw his home, and
then found the pistol he had brought home in his pack, went up
to his bedroom alone and shot himself. During the battle itself
over 400 medical personnel were admitted to the front-line
psychological units, although no other record remains of who
they were, what their symptoms were or how long they stayed
there.[1] What we do know, now as then, is that military medical
service is every bit as challenging physically and personally as
military service itself. There are thoughtful researchers doing
work to understand what the outcomes of these challenges are,
but their findings aren't likely to be in for a while, so in the
meantime here are some of my observations, made between
December 2014 and November 2016, as I talked to my medical
friends and colleagues while I was writing this book.

Medics found many different ways to cope while they were
actually in Afghanistan. One way they met the challenge was
with time and space they claimed as their own: pizza night at

the padre's, and building a defiant garden, and walking the sniffer dogs, and games, and running around the camp roads until their lungs burned and all they could do was sleep. There were the Bastion Bakers: an emergency physician, two surgeons and two anaesthetists who went into the camp kitchens in the afternoons when they weren't needed (the kitchens or the medics) and baked bread. They got really good at it – specialist ingredients sent from home, new recipes tried – Focaccia Fridays and a sourdough loaf, whose starter was taken back to the UK with its owner and was still breeding bread in 2014.[2] Good for the bakers, good for the medics who stood and ate what they had baked, something very old and helpful to humans in breaking bread together.

All of it, side-by-side therapy, watching for each other. The American surgeon who treated the Afghan children at Bastion remembered this in particular:

> Whenever the person I was entrusted to treat out there died from their wounds, I'll admit it, it hurt, and as soon as I could I would need to step outside in order to catch my breath and have my space. I did not lose a single person who could have been saved, as busy as we sometimes got I never felt panicked, but after each patient who died I got this feeling [...] I think we all got it. I expect we all got it.
>
> Later, afterwards, we all would hang together and check on one another in the little ways that really mattered, eating together, talking, finding out if the other person was alright, finding things to laugh about, exercising. It was all we could do, but it mattered and it made the difference.[3]

Some things helped some medics more than others. The repatriation ceremonies, for instance. Standing out in the open, hearing the padre lead a service for the dead. Seeing the absolute precision of the ceremony, no matter how hard the wind was blowing or the rain soaking through their uniform, unflinching, seeing the coffin taken away to the aircraft they had flown in on surrounded by living soldiers, for a journey home alone. One of the surgeons written about in this book went to every single repatriation ceremony held at Bastion while he was there, and there were many. He considered it the least he could do, part of his work. Another, who certified the dead in the cool dark of the mortuary tent, went to only one; one was enough, no more. His time could be better spent.

The junior trauma surgeon went back to his tent and wrote the diaries that became such an important primary source for this book. He wrote, no matter how tired he was, whenever he had a break, once sitting in the sunshine outside the NAAFI canteen, with a huge mug of tea. He wrote quickly, and clearly and with no spelling mistakes or crossings out. It flowed out of him, page after page, filling volumes of red exercise books that he brought with him from home specially for the purpose. He'd begun diaries when he was in Iraq. They told of fear, and on the front page had little drawings of a mortar every time one landed close enough to him to be a near miss (forty-six in all). There was almost no fear at Bastion. The occasional rocket landed, but far away in the camp, and he never had to take cover under a hospital bed. He wrote of things that medical officers have so often written of, whatever or when-ever the war. Of the weather, and of letters from home, and of nature somehow finding a way into their lives. Of his frus-tration with newly arrived officers who thought they could tinker with a system that already worked, of friends coming and going, but mostly of the work. No lists, just paragraphs of narrative of surgery, a conversation in his head:

> Both operating tables stayed open pretty much con-stantly. GSW abdo, fragmentation to the face, blast to lung, unilateral traumatic amputations, bilateral lower limb amputations, GSW leg, GSW knee, fragmenta-tion abdo, hand trauma, finger trauma, fragmentation

buttock, fragmentation upper limb … these are the cases
I can remember. There were more.

He remembered most of the individual procedures but
very few of the individuals. It surprises him today when he
meets someone who was one of his patients in the trauma bay
or chilly operating theatre at Bastion, but it doesn't bother him
particularly. He had been very angry, for years after Iraq, but
after Afghanistan he became trauma registrar at Birmingham
and then came to Imperial to research heterotopic ossification,
which is how I met him. He thinks that working to understand
the science of the severe casualty he treated back at Bastion has
helped him be less angry, to unpack the meaning of his own
experiences, to decompress.

Decompression is a technical term used by the military
for a scheduled period immediately after deployment where
personnel are given time to unwind physically and mentally.
Everyone coming back from Afghanistan, including most
of the medics, stopped over in Cyprus for around thirty-six
hours,

> in a friendly environment that allows you time to start
> 'winding down' prior to rejoining friends and family in
> the UK. It provides time to talk through your memor-
> ies with friends and colleagues who have shared similar
> experiences to your own.[4]

Decompression works for soldiers, who travelled and decom-
pressed together as a formed unit – on the beach, at the show in
the evening, on the deckchairs by the pool. But medics travelled
singly, alone in the crowd. And once the crowd discovered who
they were, they wanted to ask them hard questions about their
mates who didn't make it home, or who went home in CCAST
weeks ago, and what happened to them in detail, what they'd
done – how many amputations, how did they go, why did he
die? So no decompression for them, just being forced to relive

over and over in detail what they had been doing: no jokes, back to their surgeon voices, dragging it all back up again in the queue for food, on the beach, in the shared camp bathrooms. Often not decompression, only more compression.

The hand surgeon remembers not only every individual procedure he did but every individual he did them to, and it was a lot because with his beep, 'Doe, a Deer', he went to every single trauma call, and many considered him the hardest-working man in Bastion. For him, 'you are always linked once you've removed someone's limb'. Every single trauma call, one day after another, and he knew he had to develop some kind of coping strategy, some kind of resilience. So he told me that each day he put all the memories he accumulated at Bastion in a box in his head, and closed the lid on them tightly and didn't think about them until he got home, and by the time he had finished his second tour, the box was pretty full. At the same time, looking back, for him and for most of the surgeons there was a sense of satisfaction, of a job mostly well done, of being lucky to have seen it all and been part of something so extraordinary and not been found wanting, and a sense that they might never be quite as important, as necessary, as this again, at least professionally.[5] That sense helped them then and helps them now.

Back home and back to work. The hand surgeon works at a London hospital with a huge trauma unit, and every time, every single time, he hears a helicopter there's the same knot in his stomach that he had at Bastion, hearing MERT arrive at Nightingale, 'Doe, a Deer', waiting behind the yellow line for the call. He too was angry for a long time after he came back from his second tour, and when he discussed a third with his family, they said no, absolutely not. And so, knowing he would not return, he started to unpack the box in his memory, starting with the difficult cases, the failures. Unpack the deaths. The time when he had to call a halt and stop the team who were sure life would somehow come back from where it had been lost with only a few minutes' more work. The moment he examined a child burned all over except for a patch of undamaged skin under one of her arms and who died because there was nothing at all that he or anyone else could do for her except relieve her pain.

He considers it part of his responsibility to seek out the patients whose hands he amputated, to see how they are recovering, to 'make an apology' (his own words). He went to the military ward at Birmingham one day to meet the soldier whose hand he had really tried to save, fixation error, but could not. He started by introducing himself: 'I was part of your operating team at Bastion. Is there anything you want to know?' The soldier was pleased to see him, sat up in bed and smiled, but kept the stump of his arm covered with a sheet. His girlfriend and parents were in the room with them, and so somehow the hand surgeon never got to say what he wanted: 'I'm sorry I had to take your hand off.' He still hasn't, even though he knows the patient well now because their paths cross professionally, and the patient knows who he is and what he did. He's waiting for his chance to ask about it, and that's when he'll be able to make his apology (and the patient will probably be puzzled that he needs to do so at all because, after all, as a result of his surgery he didn't die). At the medical school where we both work he teaches the two hand cases he described for me in this book, with a PowerPoint presentation and photographs, and he shows each new generation of surgical residents what success and failure really mean.

Packing and unpacking boxes of memories, trying to make sense, reordering. That's what the American surgeon calls it.

It's not PTSD – it's different [...] I've looked it up and it doesn't quite fit [...] whatever version of PTS that I might have right now it does not feel like a 'Disorder' I don't think. Even though I get to have my issues, it feels like there is still some kind of 'Order' to them, 'PTSO', perhaps, like something necessary is going on, and my soul or psyche is busy achieving its new balance [...] This process, this PTS re-ordering, I think it's the process for how I will get back to what I was. It wouldn't make sense otherwise.

Back at work, back at home. Yet how to get back home, really, knowing something has been left behind? (I would have rewritten this, but the surgeon has put it so beautifully and when I read it to other surgeons they said that is it *exactly*.) So, in his words:

> They say war is intoxicating, but it wasn't intoxicating for me. It's like the intensity and the sharpness of the experience carved deep channels in my mind, and my thoughts as they flow about their daily business easily find themselves rolling downstream into those channels [...]
>
> Since I've been back, I've been moulting, I suppose. I'm impacted but not injured. I've had up days and some down ones too [...] It's like there are these pockets of soap bubbles of overpowering emotion floating about in my life's arena, and when I'm not bopping into them and they're not bopping into me everything is fine, perfectly fine. But there you can be, marching along, doing your thing, and one of those little bubbles find you and 'pop' it bursts and for a little bit you're under its spell and you're right back in Afghanistan or more likely you're just getting emotional and tearing up for no reason. 'It's my allergies' I say as I excuse myself if there's someone around.[6]

Almost everyone I have met in writing this book has gone back to their post in the NHS or the Defence Medical Service, to medical schools or to their practices. They research, treat and teach. The anaesthetist team leader from MERT goes out regularly with the air ambulance service in their helicopter, and when he is on board, everyone learns. They remember. The DCCN was posted overseas in 2016, but her personal diary went with her, along with the annual quietness on the anniversary of the deaths of her Bastion patients.

For them all, small things can trigger big memories. One MERT medic had stains all along the edge of his canvas watch-strap where blood had seeped over his disposable gloves during a long and complicated resuscitation in the back of the helicopter. There was no cleaning the strap, and he didn't have a spare, so last thing at night and first thing every morning the blood-stains were what he saw when he put his watch on or took it off. Khaki canvas watchstraps always start him remembering. Recently I went to hear a lecture from a surgeon who had been at Bastion in all the worst years, and I put a pile of papers down in front of me that had a 9-Liner set on the top. These are visually quite distinct: laminated plastic cards, pale pink, pre-printed with a list of the information that will be needed to call down MERT, all held together on a steel ring. While the surgeon waited to start, he caught a glimpse of the 9-Liner lying in front of me and he stopped stock still, for that extra second that doesn't have much to do with time. And then he laughed, a little, and said. 'Oops, bit of a flashback there.' And I put it away, out of sight, and was sorry not to have known better.

In many cases, diaries have been replaced with photographs, endless scrolling of photographs from their mobile phones and now on their computers. Some of them look at them too much, know the images too well and should probably put them away at some point. Perhaps there should be some research on the impact of personal photo archives, a brain scan to see what happens when they look back. Many of them continue to deploy, or go and train medics in countries they once deployed in, where things have really not got any better since they left, and I worry about them, which they think is funny, but it's hard not to worry when you work in a blast injury studies centre.

When I look back through the notes I took during my interviews, it strikes me that everyone I spoke to could fit into one of two categories. Some (most) spoke from memory – well-organised narrative memory, tour by tour, case by case, giving meaning to their actions, or still seeking it, and using their time talking to advance that process. Even if they needed diaries or their photographs to remind them of details, even if it was the first time they had spoken about their experiences at length, their thoughts were ordered and their retelling was calm, reflective, self-aware. Sometimes they looked out of the window and took a few slow breaths, and then continued. Several pushed up the sleeves on their scrubs and showed me where the cutis ansorina (medical term for goosebumps) had appeared as they remembered and talked, or laughed about the sweat on the palms of their hands and from their foreheads, as their bodies still kept the score of their experiences.

Then there was a second group that I spoke to (not many), who switched into what seemed to be another personality when they talked about Afghanistan and their work there. They suddenly switched to the present tense. Short bursts of words. Pauses. Clenched fists hidden under the table. And they were unable to guide me through a linear, chronological narrative, no matter how much prompting from diaries, or journal articles or photographs. They flashed up fragments, phrases, moments – sometimes it felt like a bombardment from their past and I didn't know where to look or what to write down. Despite our friendship, their support for the work, they moved into a space where suddenly they were mystified by my attempts to order the technical experiences of combat medicine – *it can't be done, you don't understand, everything happened at once, it can't be explained, not if you weren't there, aren't there now. Emily, I don't want to be in Helmand any more.* My questions had taken them somewhere where they were not masters of their memories, and so, once I had come to understand what the difference between the two groups meant, I stopped asking them to speak about it at all, even in a roundabout way. And I took out all the material I got from them because it did not belong in a history book.

From both groups, many have made the same casual remark: *I'll deal with all of this when I retire*, and something in me hopes (if that is the right word) that this will be the case. Recently another American surgeon who served in Vietnam, working on so many injured children that he became a paediatrician on his return home, wrote of just how this happens. How, no matter how long after the event, he and his colleagues from all the wars since will always have hard questions to ask of themselves.

Older folks like me are always surprised when they become symptomatic long after the trauma has occurred. Ageing veterans are more vulnerable physically, psychologically and financially, and they have more time for reflection. When I told a Veterans Affairs psychologist that I did not think my late-in-life symptoms were related to my Vietnam experience, he smiled. 'If you really believe that you were not affected by running into a minefield, disarming a disturbed soldier while he was threatening to shoot you, and watching your patients die while you treated them in the mud and under fire – you are an idiot.'

[...] I did not realise that the intimacy of just being present when a patient died would create an existential bond that would always be remembered [...] It was likely that some decisions made using an in-the-moment survival mentality would breach our own deeply held moral beliefs. And when we revisit them, absent the drama and without the support of like-minded individuals, we know there can be no do-overs – only the do-laters that will become our challenges for the future.

If we allow ourselves to carefully examine the events and decisions that injured our moral selves and ask, 'What kind of person am I?' the answer will be very complicated.[7]

Notes

NB: All sources quoted in notes are available on publicly accessible sources apart from those where the author is given as 'anonymous' and the document is unpublished.

Introduction
1. Ewert, K., *Henry V: A Guide to the Text and Its Theatrical Life* (Basingstoke: Palgrave Macmillan, 2006), pp. 70–74.
2. Cohort: an ancient Roman military unit; a band of warriors, persons banded together especially in a common cause; a group of persons with a common statistical characteristic; in epidemiology, a group of individuals sharing a common symptom, condition or characteristic acquired at the same time and observed over time as a group.
3. Solomon, E., and Jones, S., 'Defusing the Isis bomb industry', *Financial Times,* 29 October 2016.

The War in Afghanistan: Timeline
1. MoD factsheet from 2009, cited in Ledwidge, F., *Losing Small Wars* (New Haven, CT: Yale University Press, 2011), p. 63. See also Ledwidge, F., *Investment in Blood* (New Haven, CT: Yale University Press, 2014).

1. 'Blood is the argument': The Pathophysiology of Shock
1. Hodgetts, T., Mahoney, P., and Clasper, J. (eds), *Battlefield Advanced Trauma Life Support*, Joint Services Publication 570, 5th edn (2008).

2. Scott Meenagh
1. Unlu, A., Kaya, E., Guvenc, I., et al., 'An evaluation of CAT on training military personnel: changes in application times and success rates in three successive phases', *Journal of the Royal Army Medical Corps* (*JRAMC*), 11 November 2014. Also any article found under the keyword search 'Tourniquet' in the archives of the *JRAMC*.

2. Hodgetts, T. J., 'A Revolutionary Approach to Combat Casualty Care', unpublished PhD thesis, City University of London, October 2012, p. 45.

3. Sheers, Owen, *The Two Worlds of Charlie F* (London: Faber & Faber, 2010), p. 31.

4. Hodgetts, T. J., 'A Revolutionary Approach to Combat Casualty Care', p. 68.

5. A tourniquet features in both the trauma and the psychiatric injury sections of the Science Museum's exhibition 'Wounded: Conflict, Casualties and Care' (2016–18).

6. The sound archive of Terrence Rymer in the Imperial War Museum (IWM), no. 33806, reels 1–2.

7. Evriades, D., Jefferey, S., Cubison, T., et al., 'Shaping the military wound: issues surrounding the reconstruction of injured servicemen at the RCDM', *Philosophical Transactions of the Royal Society B,* 2011; 366: pp. 219–30, p. 221.

8. NHS news archive, 'Independent review of major trauma network reveals increase in survival rates', 25 June 2013. At least three hundred unexpected survivors per year since 2012, according to the Nottingham Trauma Centre (emailed conversation with DNRC, 2017).

9. This section is adapted from Croucher, Matt, *Bulletproof* (London: Arrow Books, 2010), pp. 68–91.

10. Roberts, D., and Aldington, D., 'Why pain relief is important: the physiological response', in Mahoney, P., and Buckenmaier, C. (eds), *Combat Anaesthesia: The First 24 Hours* (Houston, TX: The Office of the Surgeon General, Borden Institute, 2015), p. 200.

11. Definition by the International Association for the Study of Pain, cited in Sanders, G., 'The physiology of acute pain', in Mahoney and Buckenmaier (eds), *Combat Anaesthesia,* p. 194.

3. Mark Ormrod (1)

1. Sheers, Owen, *Pink Mist* (London: Faber & Faber, 2013), p. 31.

2. www.markormrod.com

3. *Hamlet* (more Shakespeare), Act III, scene i: 'But that the dread of something after death,/ The undiscovered country from whose bourn/ No traveller returns.' Also used as a subtitle in a *Star Trek* film.

4. Fairweather, J., *The Good War* (London: Jonathan Cape, 2014), p. 310.

5. Fairweather, *The Good War*, p. 314.

6. Ormrod, Mark, *Man Down* (London: Corgi, 2010), p. 102.

7. This section is taken extensively from Ormrod's own remarkable accounts of his wounding in *Man Down*, pp. 15–27 and 231–9.

4. The Medical Emergency Response Team (MERT)

1. See Alex Duncan, *Sweating the Metal* (London: Hodder, 2011), pp. 20–23.
2. Kotwal, R., Howard, J., and Orman, J., 'The effect of a Golden Hour policy on the morbidity and mortality of combat casualties', *Journal of the American Medical Association (Surgery)*, 2016; 151(1): 15–24; doi: pp. 10.1001/jamasurg.2015.3104.
3. Ormrod, *Man Down*, p. 237.
4. Mahoney and Buckenmaier (eds), *Combat Anaesthesia*. All technical information for this chapter is primarily taken from this volume.
5. Taken from the testimony of Robert Moore, IWM sound archive 32509.
6. The Eyes Verbal Motor assessments are made as part of the Glasgow Coma Scale, which is commonly used to assess coma and impaired consciousness. A score for each component is given, and then a larger score. One assessment written on the knee pad was E3 V1 M6, but then the score was crossed out because the patient had died despite the work of the team. See Teasdale, G., and Jennett, B., 'Assessment of coma and impaired consciousness: a practical scale', *The Lancet*, 1974; 2: pp. 81–4.
7. Mahoney and Buckenmaier (eds), *Combat Anaesthesia,* 'Introduction'.
8. Thank you to Martin Bricknell for emphasising 'what is it like for those left behind?' in a conversation with the author at Imperial College, 24 April 2015.
9. Fairweather, *The Good War,* p. 300.
10. Terrence Rymer, IWM sound archive 33806.

5. The Deal

1. Stewart, I., Sosnov, J., Howard, J., et al., 'Retrospective analysis of long-term outcomes after combat injury: a hidden cost of war', *Circulation,* published online, 2 November 2015.
2. Stewart, Sosnov, Howard et al., 'Retrospective analysis of long-term outcomes', p. 2129.
3. Xiao, W., Mindrinos, M., Seok, J., et al., 'A genomic storm in critically injured humans', *Journal of Experimental Medicine*, 19 December 2011; 208(13): 2581–90; see Abstract.
4. Neunaber, C., Zeckey, C., Andruskow, H., et al., 'Immunomodulation in polytrauma and polymicrobial sepsis – where do we stand?', *Recent Patents on Inflammation and Allergy Drug Discovery*, January 2011; 5(1): pp. 17–25.

6. Field Hospital Camp Bastion (Bastion)

1. Unpublished diary, anonymous junior trauma surgeon.
2. Author's conversation with anonymous anaesthetist, 30 March 2015.
3. Author's conversation with anonymous anaesthetist, 30 March 2015.
4. Horne, S., and Smith, J., 'Preparation of the resuscitation room and patient reception', *JRAMC*, vol. 157, 3rd supplement, vol. 1, pp. S267–72.
5. Mahoney and Buckenmaier (eds), *Combat Anaesthesia*, p. 695.
6. Mercer, S., Fraser, S., and Via, D., in Mahoney and Buckenmaier (eds), *Combat Anaesthesia,* p. 33.
7. Tai, N., and Russell, R., 'Right turn resuscitation: FAQs', *JRAMC*, vol. 157, 3rd supplement, vol. 1, pp. S310–14.
8. Hodgetts, 'A Revolutionary Approach to Combat Casualty Care', pp. 42–4.
9. Levine, Joshua (ed.), *Forgotten Voices of the Somme* (London: Ebury Press, 2008), pp. 102–3.
10. Hoffman, Annie, *Operation Paperclip* (New York: Little, Brown, 2014), p. 214.
11. Roach, Paul, *Citizen Surgeon: A Memoir* (Chicago, IL: Bookbaby 2016), pp. 91–2.
12. Scott, R., 'Eyes', in Brooks, A., Clasper, J., Midwinter, M., et al. (eds), *Ryan's Ballistic Trauma* (London: Springer, 2011), pp. 349–60.
13. Francis, Gavin, *Adventures in Human Being* (London: Profile Wellcome Collection, 2015), p. 73, and Kirkman, E., 'Blast injury', in Brooks, Clasper, Midwinter et al., *Ryan's Ballistic Trauma*, pp. 90–98.
14. Tunnicliffe, I., and Mackenzie, B., 'Blast injuries to the lung: epidemiologies and management', *Philosophical Transactions of the Royal Society B*, 2011, p. 366.
15. Aurora, H., Rankin, S., et al., 'Blast lung injury', in *Royal British Legion Centre for Blast Injury Studies Annual Report* (London: Imperial College, 2014).

8. Bastion's Medics

1. Birds have been punctuation points for those at war for a century and perhaps beyond. See Steven Heyde, 'History as a source for innovation in landscape architecture: the First World War landscapes in Flanders', in *Studies in the History of Gardens and Designed Landscapes,* 35:3, pp. 182–97. The author cites the memories of birds during the First World War from Frank Hurley and Robert Night.
2. One of the first papers by British specialists to describe blast injury in the modern era: Edwards, D., Lane, T., Pathak, G., et al., 'Penetration of the Warrior armoured personnel carrier by shaped charge explosive

devices (IED) – emerging injury patterns', *Journal of Bone and Joint Surgery*, vol. 91-B 2009, Orthopaedic Proceedings, Supplement II.

3. Pannett, C., 'Medical aspects of modern warfare with special reference to hospital ships', *British Journal of Surgery*, 1914: pp. 470–71.

4. Pannett, 'Medical aspects of modern warfare with special reference to hospital ships'.

5. Parker, Harry, *Anatomy of a Soldier* (London: Faber & Faber, 2015), p. 2.

6. Maitland, L., Lawton, G., Baden, A., et al., 'The role of military plastic surgeons in the management of modern combat trauma: an analysis of 645 cases', *Plastic & Reconstructive Surgery*, April 2016; vol. 137: 4: 717e–724e.

7. Wood, P., Haldane, E., and Plimmer, S., 'Anaesthesia at Role 4', *JRAMC*, no. 156 (4th supplement, vol. 1): pp. S310–12, p. 310.

8. Sella, Amnon, *The Value of Human Life in Soviet Warfare* (London: Routledge, 1992), pp. 194–6, for a discussion of the role of medical provision and military morale.

9. Patsy Beesley, sound archive of the National Army Museum.

10. Hodgetts, T. J., 'Lessons from the Musgrave Park Hospital bombing', *Injury*, April 1993; 24(4): pp. 219–21.

11. Arul, G., Pugh, H., Mercer, S., et al., 'Optimising communication in the damage control resuscitation – damage control surgery sequence in major trauma management', *JRAMC*, 158(2): pp. 82–4.

12. Mahoney, P., Hodgetts, T., and Hicks, I.: 'The deployed medical director: managing the challenges of a complex trauma system', *JRAMC*, 157 (3rd supplement, vol. 1): pp. S350–56, p. 351.

13. Trauma Bay 5 had an abdominal case that had arrived earlier in the day.

14. Moy, R., 'Ethical dilemmas in providing medical care to captured persons on operations', *JRAMC* 158(1): pp. 6–9.

15. Duncan, *Sweating the Metal*, pp. 194–6.

16. Hodgetts, T. J., 'Sniffer Dogs', unpublished poem.

17. Helphand, Kenneth, *Defiant Gardens* (San Antonio, TX: Trinity University Press, 2006), p. 234.

18. Helphand, *Defiant Gardens*, conclusions.

19. *Trauma at War*, presented by Kevin Fong, BBC Radio 4, episode 2 (first broadcast March 2014).

20. Hodgetts, T. J., 'A Premonition of Death', unpublished poem.

9. History

1. Carless, A., 'Preface' to Deane, H. E., *Gymnastic Treatment for Joint and Muscle Disabilities* (London: Hodder & Stoughton, 1918), p. 16.

2. Notes from the Medical Society of London, 'Re-education of the amputated', *The Lancet*, 3 April 1920, p. 769.

3. Actually shudder. I've seen them.

4. Huggins, G. M., 'The surgery of amputation stumps based on the experience of 2,000 cases', *The Lancet*, 28 April 1917.

5. Carless, 'Preface', p. 13.

6. See the report on 'Demonstrations: fractured femurs, facial surgery', *British Medical Journal*, 26 April 1919, pp. 528–9.

7. Please note that, because I work there, this section is primarily focused on the work of scientists and clinicians at Imperial College London, but there is a range of other universities researching the effects of severe casualty, and they can be found by the usual subject-matter searches.

8. Gay, Hannah, *The History of Imperial College London, 1907–2007* (London: Imperial College, 2007), p. 133.

9. And I'm watching.

10. Jones, E., and Wessley, S., 'Interwar', in *Shellshock to PTSD* (London: Maudsley Series, 2005).

10. Critical Care

1. No shit. Taylor, C., Hettiaratchy, S., Jeffery, S., et al., 'Contemporary approaches to definitive extremity reconstruction of military wounds', *JRAMC*, 155(4): pp. 302–7.

2. This section is drawn from Romanelli, R., Vowden, K., and Wir, D., 'Exudate management made easy', *Wounds International*, 2010; 1(2). Also, Royal College of Defence Nursing, 'Challenges of training military wounds', in *This is Defence Nursing*, RCN online publication, November 2015.

3. Hill, N., Fallowfield, J., Price. S., et al., 'Review of military nutrition', *Philosophical Transactions of the Royal Society B*, 2011, pp. 234–7. Jansen, S., Turner, S., and Johnston, A., 'Nutritional management of critically ill trauma patients in the deployed military setting', *JRAMC,* 157 (3rd supplement, vol. 1): pp. S344–9. Haenboehler, E., Williams, A., Leinhase, I., et al., 'Metabolic changes after polytrauma: an imperative for nutritional support', *World Journal of Emergency Surgery*, 2006, 1:29.

4. Exhibit 22–1, 'Potential benefits of regional anaesthesia', in Mahoney and Buckenmaier (eds), *Combat Anaesthesia,* p. 242.

5. Parker, *Anatomy of a Soldier*, p. 26.

6. Edgerod, I., and Christensen, D., 'Analysis of patient diaries in Danish ICUs: a narrative approach', *Intensive and Critical Care Nursing*, 25; 2009: pp. 268–77; 'The casualty clearing station as a working unit

in the field', *JRAMC,* 32; 1916: pp. 45–6; Thomas, J., and Bell, E., 'Lost days: diaries for military intensive care patients', *Journal of the Royal Naval Medical Service,* 97; 2011: pp. 11–15; Charon, R., 'Narrative medicine: a model for empathy, reflection, profession and trust', *JAMA,* 286; 2001, 15: pp. 1897–902; Di Gangi, S., Naretto, G., Cravero, N., et al., 'A narrative-based study on communication by family members in an intensive care unit', *Journal of Critical Care,* 2013, 28, pp. 483–9. Philips, C., 'Use of patient diaries in critical care', *Nursing Standard,* 2011, 26: pp. 34–43, p. 43. See also Mayhew, E., and McArthur, D., 'A special book kept for the purpose: writing patient diaries, a century of skill in the silence, from the Great War to Afghanistan and beyond', *Intima: A Journal of Narrative Medicine,* October 2015.

7.   Author's email exchange with RAF Emergency Nurse Sgt Nicola Blake, 14 March 2015.

11. Critical Care Air Support Team (CCAST)

1.   Mahoney and Buckenmaier (eds), *Combat Anaesthesia*, p. 398.
2.   A key source for this section is http://www.cotterrell.com/ download/4267/war-and-medicine-artists-diary
3.   Brooks, Clasper, Midwinter et al., *Ryan's Ballistic Trauma*, p. 607.
4.   http://news.bbc.co.uk/1/hi/wales/8621691.stm
5.   'Bastion: an ATC's view', *Gateway Magazine*, March 2010.
6.   See Flutter, C., Ruth, M., and Aldington, P., 'Pain management during RAF strategic aeromedical evacuations', *JRAMC,* 155(1): pp. 42–67, p. 61.
7.   Jansen, J., Turner, S., and Johnston, A., 'Nutritional management of critically ill trauma patients in the deployed military setting', *JRAMC* 157 (3rd supplement, vol. 1): pp. S344–9.
8.   Conversation with anonymous military nursing sister, 14 September 2015.
9.   Freedman, L., *The Official History of the Falkland Islands Campaign*, Government Official History series (London: Routledge, 2007), vol. 2, p. 662.
10.   Lawrence, J., and Lawrence, R., *When the Fighting Is Over: Tumbledown, A Personal Story* (London: Bloomsbury, 1988), p. 41.
11.   Lawrence and Lawrence, *When the Fighting is Over*, pp. 50–53.
12.   *The Strategic Defence Review: Defence Medical Services*, House of Commons Defence Committee, 7th Report (London: The Stationery Office, 1999), p. viii.
13.   *Defence Medical Services: A Review of the Clinical Governance of the Defence Medical Service in UK and Overseas*, Commission for

Healthcare Audit and Inspection (London: The Stationery Office, 2009), p. 13.

14. 'The experience can be stark and long-lasting. Returning to the UK after my first deployment, I shared the flight home with three critically injured British soldiers, all in induced comas, and the body of a Danish soldier killed in action. It hit me then that this flight was one of many, carrying home men and women whose lives would be changed for ever, and some who had made the ultimate sacrifice.' Prince Harry, in a speech to launch the Invictus Games in the USA, 28 October 2015. The prince was referring to a flight in March 2008 where Ben McBean, who would be a room-mate of Ormrod's at Headley, was among the seriously injured. See Ormrod, *Man Down*, pp. 35, 331.

15. Conversation with anonymous CCAST nurse, May 2015.

12. Birmingham

1. Letters from Earnest Douglas, IWM archives, quoted in Mayhew, E., *Wounded: From Battlefield to Blighty* (London: The Bodley Head, 2013).
2. Evison, M., *Death of a Soldier* (London: Biteback, 2012), p. 507, and Harnden, T., *Dead Men Risen* (London: Quercus, 2011), pp. 369–10.
3. Ormrod, *Man Down,* p. 240.
4. Nutbeam, T., and Keene, D., 'Critical care management: the patient with ballistic trauma', in Brookes, Clasper, Midwinter et al., *Ryan's Ballistic Trauma*, p. 626.
5. Dutton, C., 'Critical care nursing at role four', in Brookes, Clasper, Midwinter et al., *Ryan's Ballistic Trauma*, p. 630.

13. The Duty Critical Care Nurse

1. Email correspondence with anonymous military nursing sister who conceived the DCCN role, 9 June 2015.
2. Ormrod, *Man Down*, p. 243.
3. Wood, S., and Winters, M., 'Care of the intubated emergency department patient', *Journal of Emergency Medicine,* 2011; 40(4): pp. 419–27.
4. Conversation with Edward Spurrier, orthopaedic surgeon at Birmingham, 2011.
5. See Jardeleza, T., 'Intensive care unit sedation in the trauma patient', in Mahoney and Buckenmaier (eds), *Combat Anaesthesia*, pp. 359–70.
6. Jardeleza, 'Intensive care unit sedation in the trauma patient', p. 361.
7. The process of agitated waking by soldiers in Birmingham is dramatically re-enacted in Owen Sheers's play *The Two Worlds of*

Charlie F. The play draws directly on the experience of the wounded for its material, and the parts of casualties were played by former servicemen and -women. See http://www.charlie-f.com/about.php

8. Davies, P., Scott, T., Dutton, C., et al., 'Intensive care follow-up in UK military casualties: a one-year pilot', *Journal of the Intensive Care Society*, 15(2), April 2014: pp. 112–16.

9. Berney, S., 'Physiotherapy in critical care in Australia', in *Cardiopulmonary Physical Therapy Journal*, 23(1); March 2012: p. 19.

10. Schweickert W. D., Pohlman, M. C., Pohlman, A., et al., 'Early physical and occupational therapy in mechanically ventilated critically ill patients: a randomised control trial', *The Lancet*, 2009, 10: p. 1016.

11. Millett, R., 'Structured rehabilitation within critical care', in *Critical Response: Queen Elizabeth Hospital Birmingham's Critical Care Physiotherapy Team*, Chartered Society of Physiotherapy, *Frontline* article, published online, 1 January 2014. See also McWilliams, D., and Pantelides, K., 'Does physiotherapy led early mobilisation affect length of stay in ICU?', *Journal of the Association of Chartered Physiotherapists in Respiratory Care*, 2008; 40: pp. 5–10.

12. Evriviades, D., Jeffery, S., Cubison, T., et al., 'Shaping the military wound', *Philosophical Transactions B*, 2011, p. 225, and Taylor, C., Hettiaratchy, S., Jeffery, S., et al., 'Contemporary approaches to definitive extremity reconstruction of wounds', *JRAMC*, 155(4): pp. 302–7, p. 306.

13. Taylor, Hettiaratchy, Jeffery, et al., 'Contemporary approaches to definitive extremity reconstruction of wounds', p. 305.

14. Jeffery, S., and Porter, K., 'Role four and reconstruction', in Brookes, Clasper, Midwinter et al., *Ryan's Ballistic Trauma*, p. 667.

15. Metcalfe, J., Grimer, R., and Eiser, C., 'Orthopaedic protocols for hemipelvectomy', *Journal of Bone and Joint Surgery*, 2003, vol. 85: pp. 1–50.

16. Devonport, L., Edwards, D., Edwards, C., et al., 'Evolution of the Role 4 UK military pain service', *JRAMC* 156 (supplement 1), p. 403.

17. Elaine Scarry's classic *The Body in Pain* (Oxford: Oxford University Press, 1985).

18. http://www.who.int/cancer/palliative/painladder/en/

19. Davies, P., Scott, T., Dutton, C., et al., 'Intensive care follow-up in UK military casualties: a one-year pilot'.

20. Scott Meenagh's patient diary, entry for 25 January 2011, 2020 hrs.

14. Mark Ormrod (3)

1. Ormrod, *Man Down*, pp. 244–60, for this section. The RAF's burned aircrew formed themselves into The Guinea Pig Club,

whose membership was extremely exclusive, and no one cared to pay membership voluntarily. See Mayhew, E., *The Reconstruction of Warriors* (London: Greenhill, 2004).

2.   Tallis, R., *The Hand* (Edinburgh: Edinburgh University Press, 2003), pp. 90–92.

3.   'For like a hectic in my blood he rages,
     And thou must cure me: till I know it's done
     How'er my haps, my joys were ne'er begun.'
     Claudius, in *Hamlet*, Act IV, scene iii.

4.   Kucisec-Tepes, N., Bejuk, D., and Kosuta, D., 'Characteristics of war wound infection', *Acta Medica Croatica,* September 2006; 60(4): pp. 353–63.

5.   Sheers, *Pink Mist*, p. 51.

6.   BBC Radio Wiltshire interview with Jon Le Galloudec by Ashley Heath, recorded at Tedworth House, June 2014 for *The People's War*, BBC First World War centenary commemoration.

7.   See Taylor, Hettiaratchy, Jeffery et al., 'Contemporary approaches to definitive extremity reconstruction of wounds', p. 306, and Pfaller, M., Pappas, P., and Wingard, J., 'Invasive fungal pathogens: current epidemiological trends', *Clinical Infectious Diseases*, 2006; 43 (supplement 1): pp. S3–14. See also Parker, *Anatomy of a Soldier*, p. 58.

8.   Jones, C., Chinery, J., England, K., et al., 'Critical Care at Role 4', *JRAMC*, December 2010; 156 (4th supplement, vol. 1): pp. 342–8, p. 347.

9.   See Wong, J., March, D., Abu-Sitta, G., et al., 'Biological foreign body implantation in victims of the London July 7th suicide bombings', *The Journal of Trauma*, 2006; 60(2): pp. 402–4. Also Patel, H., Dryden, S., Gupta, A., et al., 'Human body projectiles implantation in victims of suicide bombings and implications for health and emergency care providers: the 7/7 experience', *Annals of the Royal College of Surgeons of England*, 2012; 94(5): pp. 313–17.

10. Halachev, M., Chan, J., Constantinidou, C., et al., 'Genomic epidemiology of a protracted hospital outbreak caused by multidrug-resistant Acinetobacter baumannii in Birmingham England', *Genome Medicine*, 20 November 2014; 6(11): p. 70.

11. Ormrod, *Man Down*, pp. 257–8.

12. Ormrod, *Man Down*, pp. 263–4.

13. 'The casualty clearing station as a working unit in the field', *JRAMC*, 32, 1916, p. 45.

14. The correspondence of Captain Charles McKerrow and others to his wife, Jean, the archives of the Imperial War Museum: 93/20/1, p. 285.

15. Mark Ormrod (4)

1. Black Dog, 'The Great Leveller', in *Enduring Freedom* (Brighton: FireStep Publishing, 2011), p. 41.
2. Ormrod, *Man Down*, p. 267.

16. Rehabilitation: Headley Court

1. Jones, R., report on a lecture to the Hunterian Society of London, *The Lancet*, 12 January 1918, pp. 59–61.
2. For the definitive history of the development of modern orthopaedics, see Cooter, R., *Surgery and Society in Peace and War* (London: Palgrave Macmillan, 1993).
3. Deane, H., *Gymnastic Treatment for Joints and Muscle Disabilities* (Oxford: Oxford University Press, 1918), p. 13.
4. Deane, *Gymnastic Treatment for Joints and Muscle Disabilities*, p. 13.
5. Etherington, J., 'Conflict rehabilitation', in Brookes, Clasper, Midwinter et al. (eds), *Ryan's Ballistic Trauma*, pp. 669–90.
6. This section, and this set of quotations, from Etherington, 'Conflict rehabilitation', pp. 669–90.
7. David Henson, lecture at Imperial College, 1 June 2016.

17. Sockets and Stumps

1. See http://www.channel4.com/programmes/were-the-superhumans
2. Guyatt, M., 'Better legs: artificial limbs for British veterans of the First World War', *Journal of Design History*, 2001, 14(4): pp. 307–25.
3. Artists of the Italian Renaissance, not Ninja Turtles.
4. Harry Parker took particular care with the way he communicated with his prosthetist and physios, explaining in close, personal detail how his new limbs were working for him, and you can see how well this translated into his fictional account of a wounding, in *Anatomy of a Soldier*. Author's conversation with Harry Parker, 16 February 2016.
5. This section is drawn from Gillian Conway's excellent presentation at Imperial College during the Rehab Research Seminar series, 3 February 2016.
6. McGregor, A., Hopkins, M., et al., 'Blast injury rehabilitation', *Royal British Legion Centre for Blast Injury Studies, Annual Report 2014* (London: Imperial College, 2014), p. 30.
7. Ormrod, *Man Down*, p. 305.
8. Author's conversation with Harry Parker, 16 February 2016.
9. Jones, R., 'An address on the orthopaedic outlook in military surgery', given at the Hunterian Society, Royal College of Surgeons, 2 January 1918.

10. http://www.findabetterway.org.uk/news/
    fabw-funded-surgical-course-huge-success/
11. Ormrod, *Man Down*, pp. 308–10.

18. Mark Ormrod (5)
1. Ormrod, 'Parenting with a disability', 15 September 2015, www.
   markormrod.com
2. Ormrod, *Man Down*, p. 320.

19. A Short History of Headley Court and Its Garden (neither of which is as old as it looks)
1. See Gruber von Arni, E., *Justice to the Maimed Soldier: Nursing and Medical Care for Sick and Wounded Soldiers and their Families in the English Civil War and Interregnum* (London: Routledge, 2001).
2. http://www.epsomandewellhistoryexplorer.org.uk/Weather.pdf
3. Land Use Consultants, 'Historical Development', in *Headley Court Development Plan,* section 2.0, pp. 1–11 (author's own copy).
4. Hodgson Burnett, Frances, *The Secret Garden* (London: Vintage Classics, 2012), p. 281.
5. http://www.londonskateparks.co.uk/skateparks/southbank/

20. Sockets and Stumps and Pain
1. Jon Kendrew, lecture at Imperial College, London, 1 June 2016.
2. 'The problem of the disabled soldier', editorial in *The Lancet*, 18 November 1916, pp. 867–8.
3. Jones, R., Hunterian Society lecture on wartime orthopaedic surgery, reprinted in *The Lancet,* 12 January 1918, pp. 59–61.
4. Hsu, E., and Cohen, S., 'Post-amputation pain: epidemiology, mechanisms and treatment', *Journal of Pain Research*, 2013; 6: pp. 121–36.
5. Aldington, D., Small, C., Edwards, D., et al., 'A survey of post-amputation pains in serving military personnel', *JRAMC*, 2014; 160: pp. 38–41.
6. Le Feuvre, P., and Aldington, D., 'Know pain, know gain', *JRAMC,* 2014; 160: pp. 16–21.
7. See Edwards, D., Mayhew, E., and Rice, A., '"Doomed to go in company with miserable pain": surgical recognition and treatment of amputation-related pain on the Western Front during World War One', *The Lancet*, 8 November 2014; 384: pp. 1715–19.
8. Devonport, Edwards et al., 'Evolution of the Role 4 UK military pain service', p. 403.
9. Thank you to Peter Berg and the writers of the film *Deepwater Horizon* (Summit Entertainment et al.) for that one.

21. PTSD (Trauma Reaction)

1. This section on the planting of the walled garden is taken from Thomas Meenagh's own unpublished record, 'The Headley Court Garden'.

2. William Shakespeare, *Troilus and Cressida,* Act III, scene iii, line 175.

3. Miller, Clarence, 'On A Man for All Seasons', *Thomas More Studies* (1), 2006, pp. 27–9, and *The Complete Works of St Thomas More* (New Haven, CT: Yale University Press, 1967–93). Miller clarifies that the original phrase 'A man for all seasons' is taken from Erasmus' original Latin, which precisely translates as 'a man suited to all hours, times, occasions'.

4. The student was Marie Jacobsen, who has since graduated and returned to her home town of Adelaide in Australia (email correspondence with Thomas Meenagh, October 2015).

5. This is called animal therapy. Scientists are looking at this now because it works. See Levinson, B., 'Human companion animal therapy', *Journal of Contemporary Psychotherapy,* 14(2); 1984: pp. 131–44, and Fine, A., *Handbook on Animal Assisted Therapy* (London: Academic Press, 2010).

6. Poultry farming was used in the aftermath of the First World War as part of the rehabilitation and retraining of casualties. There was a poultry farm in Welwyn Garden City where casualties learned the skills required and could keep a small flock domestically as a potential source of income. Thank you to Jenna Stevens-Smith, whose grandfather William Lane was one of them.

7. Wilson, E., *Biophilia* (Cambridge, MA: Harvard University Press, 1990), p. 101.

8. Jeff Goldblum as chaos theory specialist Ian Malcolm in the film *Jurassic Park.*

9. For the benefits of horticultural therapy see: Mitchell, R., Astell-Burt, T., and Richardson, E. A., 'A comparison of green space indicators for epidemiological research', in *Journal of Epidemiology and Community Health*, October 2011; 65: pp. 853–8; Lewis, C., 'Human health and well-being: the psychological, physiological, and sociological effects of plants on people', *Acta Horticultura*, 1995; 391: pp. 31–40; Wichrowski, M., Whiteson, J., Haas F., et al., 'Effects of horticultural therapy on mood and heart rate in patients participating in an inpatient cardiopulmonary rehabilitation program', *Journal of Cardiopulmonary Rehabilitation,* 2005, 25(5): pp. 270–74; Van Den Berg, A., and Custers, M., 'Gardening promotes neuroendocrine and affective restoration from stress', *Journal of Health Psychology*, January 2011; 16: pp. 3–11; Hartig, T., Evans, G., Jamner, L. D., et al. 'Tracking restoration in

natural and urban field settings', *Journal of Environmental Psychology*, 2003; 23: pp. 109–23; Kaplan, R., and Kaplan, S., 'Preference, restoration, and meaningful action in the context of nearby nature', in Bartlett, P. F. (ed.), *Urban Place: Reconnecting with the Natural World* (Cambridge, MA: The MIT Press, 2005), pp. 271–98; Hartig, T., and Cooper Marcus, C., 'Healing gardens: places for nature in health care', *The Lancet*, 2006; 368: pp. S36–7; Pretty, J., Peacock, J., Sellens, M., et al., 'The mental and physical health outcomes of green exercise', *International Journal of Environmental Health Research*, 2005; 15(5): pp. 319–37; Barton, H., and Grant, M., 'A health map for the local human habitat', *Journal of the Royal Society for the Promotion of Health*, 2006; 126(6): pp. 252–3; Burls, A., 'People and green spaces: promoting public health and mental well-being through ecotherapy', *Journal of Public Mental Health*, 2007; 6(3): pp. 24–39; Gerlach-Spriggs, N., and Healy, V., 'The therapeutic garden: a definition', *ASLA Healthcare and Therapeutic Design Newsletter*, 2010 (online); and Greenberg, N., Iversen, A., Hull, L., et al., 'Getting a peace of the action: measures of post traumatic stress in UK military peacekeepers', *Journal of the Royal Society of Medicine*, February 2008; 101(2): pp. 78–84. Thank you to Peter Le Feuvre, who compiled this index so I didn't have to.

10. Hickman, C., *Therapeutic Landscapes* (Manchester: Manchester University Press, 2013), and Dixon Hunt, J., *A World of Gardens* (London: Reaktion, 2012).

11. Helphand, *Defiant Gardens*, pp. 2–6.

12. Dixon Hunt, *A World of Gardens*, pp. 21 and 83–91, and Dixon Hunt, J., *Historical Ground* (London: Routledge, 2014), p. 21.

13. Fox, J., 'Conflict and consolation: British art and the First World War, 1914–1919', *Art History*, vol. 36, 2013: pp. 810–33, for details of Howard Kemp-Prosser's visionary formulation of colour therapy.

22. The Engineer: Dave Henson

1. See Craig Miller, B., *Empty Sleeves: Amputation in the Civil War South* (Athens, GA: University of Georgia Press, 2015), p. 146.

2. Guyatt, M., 'Better legs: artificial limbs for British Veterans of the First World War', *Journal of Design History,* vol. 14, no. 4, pp. 307–25, p. 321.

23. A Centre for Blast Injury Studies

1. Probably not just theoretical physics, also quantum physics, high-energy physics and engineering to build the actual machine, and this is not as funny as you think it is – there are applications to investigate time-travel possibilities. Thank you to Dr Simon Foster, solar physicist and physics outreach officer, for these insights.

2. Letter from Sir Arthur Sloggett to Sir Alfred Keogh, 9 December 1915, p. 1. Archives of King's College London. Thank you to Dr Tom David, who found this extraordinary source, recognised it for what it was and told me about it.

3. Kotwal, R., Howard, J., and Ormon, J., 'Effect of Golden Hour policy on the morbidity and mortality of combat casualties', *Journal of the American Medical Assocation (Surgery)*, 2016; 151(1): pp. 15–24. doi: 10.1001/jamasurg.2015.3014.

4. The history of how Imperial got its Blast Lab, which eventually became the TRBL Centre for Blast Injury Studies, cannot be adequately summed up in two lines, obviously. But an account of that particular history is in progress.

5. Thank you to Hari Aurora and Phil Pearce, who provided the concept of the car alarm of blast injury in the human body during their Imperial Festival lecture, May 2016.

6. Edwards, D., Lane, D., Pathak, G., et al., 'Penetration of the Warrior armoured personnel carrier by shaped charge explosive devices (IED) – emerging injury patterns', *Journal of Bone and Joint Surgery*, vol. 91-B, 2009, Orthopaedic Proceedings, Supplement II; Ramasamy, A., Harrisson, S., Clasper, J., et al., 'Injuries from roadside improvised explosive devices', *Journal of Trauma*, 65(4), 2008: pp. 910–14; Ramasamy, A., Harrison, S., Lasrado, M., et al. 'A review of casualties during the Iraqi insurgency 2006 – a British field hospital experience', *Injury*, 40 (2009): pp. 493–7.

7. Ramasamy, A., Hill, A., Masouros, S., et al., 'Evaluating the effect of vehicle modification in reducing injuries from landmine blasts: an analysis of 2212 incidents and its application for humanitarian purposes', *Accident Analysis and Prevention*, 2011; 43(2): pp. 1878–86.

8. Author's conversation with Spyros Masouros and Adam Hill, September 2015.

9. Spyros Masouros, conversation with the author, November 2015.

10. For a full round-up of all Imperial's Centre for Blast Injury Studies research programmes see Bull, A., Clasper, J., and Mahoney, P., *Blast Injury Science and Engineering: A Guide for Clinicians and Researchers* (London: Springer, 2016).

11. Ulgen, B., Brumblay, H., Yang, L. J., et al., 'Augusta Déjerine-Klumpke, M.D. (1859–1927): a historical perspective on Klumpke's palsy', *Neurosurgery*, August 2008; 63(2): pp. 359–66.

12. Edwards, D., Clasper, J., and Patel, H., 'HO in victims of the London 7/7 bombings', *JRAMC*, 5 December 2014.

13. 'Kabul attack offers a grim test to a tiny ambulance crew', *New York Times*, 21/22 April 2016.

24. Mark Ormrod (6)

1. Mark Ormrod, blog post: http://www.markormrod.com/2015/07/17/de-cluttering-organisation
2. Mark Ormrod, blog post, de-cluttering, p. 3.
3. Mark Ormrod, blog post, 'Tips for better health (part two)', 19 May 2016.

25. Sockets and Stumps and Science

1. Haufner, S., 'Considerations for development of sensing and monitoring tools to facilitate treatment and care of persons with lower limb loss: a review', *Journal of Rehabilitation Research and Development* 2014; vol. 51, no.1: 1–14, p. 3.
2. Thank you to Dr Claire Higgins for her remarkable insights in this section.
3. Claire does this sort of thing: Topouzi, H., and Higgins, C. A., 'Expression map of three distinct skin fibroblast populations isolated from human skin', 45th Annual Meeting of the European Society for Dermatological Research (Nature Publishing Group, 2015).

26. Complex Outcomes, Chronic Pain and PTSD

1. Author's conversation with Dominic Aldington, Winchester, 2015.
2. See Grichnik, K., and Ferrante, F., 'The difference between acute and chronic pain', *Mt Sinai Journal of Medicine*, May 1991; 58(3): pp. 217–20, p. 217 (abstract).
3. Stephens, R., Atkins, J., and Kingston, A., 'Swearing as a response to pain', *NeuroReport*, 2009; 20(12): pp. 1056–60.
4. Latremoliere, A., and Woolf, C., 'Central sensitization: a generator of pain hypersensitivity by central neural plasticity', *Journal of Pain*, September 2009; 10(9): pp. 895–926 (a very long article, very complicated, with the longest bibliography I've ever seen, but possibly the most important reference in this book).
5. Anything by Lorrimer Moseley and his brain team explains this process beautifully.
6. Van der Kolk, B., *The Body Keeps the Score* (London: Penguin, 2014), pp. 1–2. Thank you to Matthew Green, who drew my attention to this work, and also for his own definitive study of PTSD in the contemporary era: Green, M., *Aftershock: Fighting War, Surviving Trauma, Finding Peace* (London: Portobello, 2016). If you only read two books about pain and PTSD, make sure they are both by Steve Haines: *Trauma Is Really Strange* and *Pain Is Really Strange* (both London: Singing Dragon, 2016). From them you will understand how therapy for chronic pain and PTSD is really well done.

7. Otis, J., Keane, T., and Kerns, R., 'An examination of the relationship between chronic paiñ and post-traumatic stress disorder', *Journal of Rehabilitation Research and Development*, September/October 2003; 40(5): pp. 397–406, p. 397.

8. Risdall, J., and Menon, D., 'Traumatic brain injury', *Philosophical Transactions of the Royal Society B* (theme issue, 'Military Medicine in the 21st Century: Pushing the Boundaries of Combat Casualty Care'), 2011; 366: pp. 241–50.

9. Cassandra Jardine, interview with Robert Lawrence: 'Angry, my wife calls me Social Semtex', *Daily Telegraph,* 3 April 2007.

10. Risdall and Menon, 'Traumatic brain injury', p. 247.

11. Sofroniew, M., and Vinters, H., 'Astrocytes: biology and pathology', *Acta Neuropathologica*, January 2010, 119(1): pp. 7–35.

12. Shively, S., Horkayne-Szakaly, I., Jones, R., et al., 'Characterisation of interface astroglial scarring in the human brain after blast exposure: a post-mortem case series', *The Lancet Neurology*, published online, 9 June 2016. Professor Perl and his research are mentioned at an early stage in Mary Roach's brilliant *Grunts: The Curious Science of Humans at War* (London: Oneworld, 2016).

13. Worth, R., 'What if PTSD is more physical than psychological?', *New York Times Magazine,* 10 June 2016.

14. Shively, S., Horkayne-Szakaly, I., Perl, D., et al., 'Research in context', editorial comment on 'Characterisation of interface astroglial scarring in the human brain after blast exposure: a post-mortem case series'.

Epilogue: Medics

1. Jones, E., Thomas, A., and Ironside, S., 'Shell shock: an outcome study of a First World War "PIE" unit', *Psychological Medicine*, 2007; 37: pp. 215–23.

2. Arul, G., Bree, S., Sonka, B., et al., 'The secret lives of the Bastion Bakers', *British Medical Journal*, 349, 18 December 2014. Thank you to Alan Kay, who brought this excellent source to my attention, and to the *BMJ*'s Christmas editors for their usual deft touch with content.

3. Roach, *Citizen Surgeon*.

4. Royal Navy, *So You're Going on Decompression?* (Fleet Graphics Centre, 10/408).

5. Roach, *Citizen Surgeon*, p. 188.

6. Roach, *Citizen Surgeon*.

7. Brown, J., 'The moral matrix of wartime medicine', *Intima: A Journal of Narrative Medicine*, September 2015.

Acknowledgements

Dominic Aldington
Ben Almquist
Marie Anneberg Jensen
Hari Arora

Roderick Bailey
Spencer Barnes
Nicola Blake
Jens Brahe Pedersen
Martin Bricknell
Richard Broadbridge
Anthony Bull
Emma Burke
Peter Buxton

Sarah Cage-Brimelow
Steven Campbell
    Moore
Dilen Carpanen
Jon Clasper
Gillian Conway
David Cotterell
Jim Czarnik

Tom David
Penny Davies
Christian Dinesen
Clare Dutton

Daffyd Edwards
Stewart Emmens
Margaret Evison

Sebastian Faulks
Robert Fleming
Aimee Foster
Simon Foster
James Fox
Gavin Francis
Rupert Frere

Claire Goodall
Katie Gonzalez-Bell
Timothy
    Granville-Chapman
Matthew Green
Teresa Griffiths
Kirby Gross

Alex Haley
Christine Hallett
David Harding
Phoebe Harkins
Carson Hart
Vikki Hawkins
David Henson
Shehan Hetticharatchy
Emma Hey
Claire Higgins
Adam Hill
Timothy Hodgetts
Alison Hoffman
Matt Hopkins
Jeff Howard

Colin Hughes
Michael Hughes
Richard Hughes

Soundararajan Jagdish
Hanna Jarvis
Edgar Jones

Alan Kay
Harriet Kemp
Jon Kendrew
Russ Kotwal

Di Lamb
Peter Le Feuve
Paul Levy

David Mcarthur
Geraldine McCool
Ross Macfarlane
Alison McGregor
Peter Mahoney
Tamar Makin
Sanders Marble
Spyros Masouros
James Mayhew
Robert Mayhew
Scott Meenagh
Thomas Meenagh
Mungo Melvin
Julia Midgeley
Brian Miller

Simon Miller

Tim Nicholson Roberts

Mark Ormrod

Harry Parker
Duncan Parkhouse
Phil Pearce
Andrew Phillips
Maryam Philpott
Laura Piddock
Aarathi Prasad
Duncan Precious
Kate Pryor
Owen Pritchard

Ian Radcliffe
Sara Rankin
Dominic Reid

Andrew Rice
Rory Rickard
Dan Roberts
William Rollo
Jane Rosen
Paul Roach
Martin Ruth

Robert Schroter
Peter Scott
Julie Sessions
Anna Sharrock
Owen Shears
Kate Sherman
Helen Singh
Ed Spurrier
Rachel Staples
William Statz

Jenna Stevens-Smith
Ian Stewart
Dan Stinner
Alexander Stoddart
Christopher Stoltz

Neil Taylor
Jason Thomas
Luke Thompson

David Vassalo

Lorraine Ward
Claire Webster
David Wiseman
Emma Willis
Mark Wyldebore

A Note on the Photographs

There is no conventional plate section in *A Heavy Reckoning*. Instead, images which represent the significant themes of the book are compiled into a photo-essay, accompanied by short phrases matched to the text. The visuals have been drawn from the work of David Cotterrell and Rupert Frere.

David Cotterrell is an installation artist working across media and technologies to explore the social and political tendencies of a world at once shared and divided. In 2007, he went to Afghanistan on a war artist commission from Wellcome Collection, undertaking a residency with the Joint Forces Medical Group in Helmand Province. When he returned he sought to develop work that responded to the extraordinary experience of witnessing individuals striving to support others to maintain an elite level of health, while preparing for the possibility of treating them again for the most profound threats to their mental and physical survival. David's subsequent work *Theatre* was the centerpiece of the *War and Medicine* exhibition held at Wellcome Collection in 2008.

Staff Sergeant Rupert Frere is a British Army Photographer. The Army's photographic branch is responsible for all photography in the Army. Wherever the Army is on operational duties a photographer accompanies them to provide images for the Defence Imagery Archive, for release to the press, or for intelligence purposes. Rupert first deployed to Helmand in 2009 as part of a combat camera team. He went for a second tour in 2010 as the Task Force Helmand photographer with 16 Air Assault Brigade. Rupert describes the difference between a war photographer and an army photographer thus: army photographers carry a weapons system as well as a camera. On occasion they make a choice between capturing the action or becoming part of it. Sometimes they do both.

Photo credits
David Cotterrell: 1, 6 (bottom); Rupert Frere: 2 top), 2(bottom), 3 (top), 3 (bottom), 4 (top), 4 (bottom), 5, 6 (top), 7 (top), 7 (bottom), 8 (bottom); Mark Ormrod: 8 (top left); Scott Meenagh: 8 (top right).

INDEX

MIST(AT) REPORT

This additional MIST(AT) REPORT can be detached
and back loaded with the casualty

Do not delay launch of MEDEVAC – supply further information once available:

Zap Number	If Known			
				e.g. TA2324

M	**Mechanism of Injury** (And at what time if known)	(M)		(Time: ....)	
I	**Injury or Illness Sustained**	(I)			
	Symptoms and Vital Signs	(S)			
S	C – Catastrophic Bleeding A – Airway B – Breathing C – Pulse Rate D – Conscious / Unconscious E – Other Signs	Time .... C ...... A ...... B ...... C ...... D ...... E	Time .... C ...... A ...... B ...... C ...... D ...... E	Time .... C ...... A ...... B ...... C ...... D ...... E	
T	**Treatment Given** (e.g. Tourniquet and time applied, morphine)	(T)			
A	**Age of the casualty** (Adult / Child at least)				
T	**Time of wounding**				

Notes:
1. Specify if critical medical supplies are needed to be brought in with MEDEVAC.
2. '9-Line' is not used for requests to move casualties who are killed in action (KIA) at the scene.

AC71936.ADR002493   AUTHORITY: LXC, DLW - SEP 13